OVERCOME
INCONTINENCE

Practical help and encouragement for all who suffer from a
bladder control problem. A unique three-month programme
that could revolutionize your life.

'Our doubts are traitors, and make us lose the good we oft might win, by fearing to attempt.'   William Shakespeare
– Measure for Measure, I, iv.

OVERCOME INCONTINENCE

A simple self-help guide

Dr Richard J. Millard

Thorsons
An Imprint of HarperCollins*Publishers*

Thorsons
An Imprint of HarperCollins*Publishers*
77–85 Fulham Palace Road,
Hammersmith, London W6 8JB

Published by Thorsons as
Overcoming Urinary Incontinence 1988
This edition 1993
Original Australian edition published as *Bladder Control*
by Williams and Wilkins and Associates Pty Limited,
404 Sydney Road, Balgowlah, NSW 2093, Australia
10   9   8   7   6   5   4   3   2   1

Richard J. Millard asserts the moral right to
be identified as the author of this work

A catalogue record for this book
is available from the British Library

ISBN 0 7225 2937 6

Printed in Great Britain by
HarperCollinsManufacturing Glasgow

*This manual is dedicated to my patients from whom I have
learned so much.*

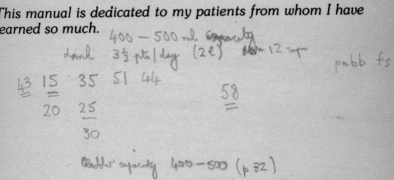

Contents

Acknowledgements

The author gratefully acknowledges the encouragement he has received from his colleagues Professor G. F. Murnaghan and Dr R. H. Farnsworth during the development of this training programme, and Pauline Chiarelli who inspired it. Acknowledgement is also made of the help of the nursing staff of the Training Unit of The Prince Henry Hospital, particularly Sister Margaret Neverly and Sister Dorothy Wheeler who assisted in the evolution of these exercise programmes into an effective treatment regimen.

Introduction

Urinary incontinence is the involuntary loss or escape of urine from the bladder. Such loss of urine can vary enormously in amount — from a 'drip' to a 'flood' — and in frequency — from occasional to many times a day. Incontinence (or leakage) is a common and distressing condition. Studies in the United Kingdom, the United States and Australia have shown an incidence of the disorder amongst their populations of about 6%. Women are 7 to 8 times more likely to be afflicted than men. A great many more people experience occasional 'accidents' with involuntary loss of small amounts of urine. Surveys have shown that 54% of women have experienced some loss of bladder control at some time in their adult life. So you are not alone in having an incontinence problem.

Urinary incontinence can be a humiliating experience. Otherwise healthy individuals suffer the indignity of embarrassing accidents in business, family and social situations. Severe degrees of incontinence can affect every aspect of a person's life. Fear and shame may lead to depression, anxiety and loss of self-confidence and self-esteem. Some people give up completely and become housebound. Many sufferers are too embarrassed to talk about their problem, even to their doctors.

This manual has been written to help those with a bladder control problem to overcome their disability. The exercises described here may completely cure you or significantly improve your control and bladder function. The advice given is based on the author's experience gained from seeing thousands of people with the problem. However, it should be stressed from the outset that only by doing the exercises properly, regularly and intelligently will you be able to benefit. The exercise programme will also help those who wish to improve their pelvic floor muscles in order to prevent themselves from developing a problem in the future and should form part of antenatal or postnatal exercise programmes.

How to Use this Manual

This manual has four main sections. The first section deals with the types and causes of incontinence and contains general advice and information. Whatever your problem you should read this section first. The second section contains a complete programme of exercises for the pelvic floor muscles and the muscles of bladder control. The third section deals with bladder training for those having trouble holding their urine for more than a short time. The fourth section contains advice for those with other incontinence problems.

If you have a bladder control problem you will need to read and work through the pelvic floor exercise programme in the second section. Some people will also need to follow the bladder training programme in the third section of the manual. It is made clear in the text which people would benefit from doing bladder training as well as the pelvic floor programme. Generally speaking, anyone with an incontinence problem will benefit from the exercises in section two, so this is where you should start.

The pelvic floor exercise programme is divided into 3 stages: preparatory exercises; basic exercise programme; and stress-specific exercises.

In order to complete the full course you will need to work through all 3 stages in turn. **Do not** proceed to a more advanced exercise until you have mastered, and made progress with, all the earlier exercises. Always keep in mind where the muscles are and what they are meant to do.

Because the majority of people who suffer from incontinence are female, much of the text of this manual is directed at women. Men should not be put off by this. The pelvic floor exercises and bladder training programmes are equally effective in restoring urinary control in men as they are in women. Men should take more care to ensure that they are using the correct muscles and it is well worth their while to study the relevant preparatory exercises carefully before proceeding further.

About 70% of the men and women who have undertaken this course of exercises have achieved satisfactory urinary control and avoided surgery. It is equally effective in those who have had previously unsuccessful surgery for their leakage problem, and at any age. There is therefore a good chance that it will help you too. No part of the programme is claimed to be original; most elements of the course have been around for years, so you can be assured that it is a tried and trusted method of treatment.

You are advised to read through the entire manual quickly at first just to gather a complete picture of the programme from start to finish. Then read it again slowly, making sure that you **fully understand every step.** As you get into the exercise programme, keep the manual handy and refer to it often to make certain that at every stage you are sure of what it is that you should be doing, and what to aim for next. Don't get impatient: slow, steady progress is what you should aim for. You should not expect to improve overnight. Keep a record of your progress at the end of each week on the chart on page 51 of the manual.

The more you know about the control of the bladder and the muscles of the pelvic floor the better equipped you will be to fight your problem. Start then by learning about the muscles and how they control the bladder. If you understand where they are in your body and what their actions are, you are more likely to use your muscles properly. Refer to the figures as you read about the pelvic floor muscles and the sphincter muscles and as you do the preparatory exercises. If you are unsure about the meaning of a word in the text look it up in the glossary before proceeding.

Section One

About Incontinence

Understanding the Urinary System

A thorough understanding of incontinence is the key to success and begins with an explanation of the urinary tract and the muscles involved in bladder control.

Urine is produced by the two kidneys which are situated in each loin. Their job is to filter the blood passing through them. Water and dissolved salts and other substances pass through the filter system, but some of these are reabsorbed in other parts of the kidney, leaving water and waste products to be eliminated in the final urine produced. The healthy adult produces about 1500ml (3 pints) of urine each full day, but there is considerable variation from day to day. The amount of urine produced depends upon the fluid intake of the individual and the amount of fluid lost in imperceptible evaporation from the breath and the skin, and by overt sweating, as well as fluid lost in the bowel motions.

The urine which is produced by the kidneys flows down two supple muscular tubes, called ureters, into the bladder. Valves at the lower end of the ureters prevent reflux of urine from the bladder back into the ureter when the bladder contracts to empty. Urine is stored in the bladder at low pressure and without voluntary effort until such time as it is convenient to urinate, at which time the urine is propelled down the urethra (or waterpipe) to the exterior by contraction of the bladder. The normal bladder holds between 400 and 500ml (20 and 25fl oz) of urine and empties 4 to 6 times each day.

Urine can only escape from the bladder, where it is stored, when the pressure inside the bladder is higher than the pressure which compresses the urethra and tends to keep it closed. In normal individuals this only occurs when the bladder contracts to empty in the voluntary act of urination (voiding). Normally, the urethra is kept adequately closed throughout the remainder of the time by muscles which encircle the urethra, compressing it to prevent leakage. These are the **sphincter muscles.**

If, for any reason, the sphincter muscles are weak, urine can leak out of the bladder when the pressure inside it is increased –

for example when a cough or sneeze causes sudden compression of the bladder. Leakage of urine under these circumstances is called stress incontinence and affects approximately 20% of adult women. It is particularly common in pregnant women, those who have had 4 or more children, and at the time of the menopause. Because it is caused by sphincter weakness, it is amenable to correction by exercises which strengthen these muscles.

The Pelvic Floor Muscles

The pelvic floor muscles span the gap between the rigid bony walls of the human pelvis like a hammock. They support not only the pelvic organs – bladder, uterus and rectum – but also, in the standing position, the entire abdominal contents.

The outlet from the bladder, called the urethra, is surrounded by muscles which are derived, in part, from the pelvic floor muscles. Similarly derived muscles surround the anus or 'back passage'. In both cases the muscles around these outlets from the body are separate from the true pelvic floor muscles, **the levators,** and are somewhat different in character. They are the sphincter muscles. Their job is to act like control valves to prevent leakage from the bladder and bowel.

In women, the pelvic floor, in addition to its role in supporting the pelvic and abdominal contents, has another important function. During childbirth it acts as a guide for the head of the baby, turning it and directing it towards the birth canal and vagina. At a later stage in the delivery, these same pelvic floor muscles are considerably stretched as the baby's head and body pass through to the outside. The bigger the baby's head, the more stretching must occur. If the delivery is very rapid the muscles may be torn, bruised and injured. The more babies, the greater are the chances of damage to the pelvic floor musculature. In addition, partial damage to the nerve supply of the muscles can occur during childbirth and results in further weakness.

Birth trauma of this kind, and changes in the muscles secondary to the menopause and ageing, are the commonest causes of pelvic floor and sphincter weakness which cause urinary incontinence. Once there is weakness in these control mechanisms, hormonal changes such as occur at period time can exacerbate the leakage problem. Obesity aggravates the problem all the time. For example, 10kg of excess weight is like carrying two house bricks around within you all day and night. A great deal of this extra weight rests on the pelvic floor, stretching and weakening it even more.

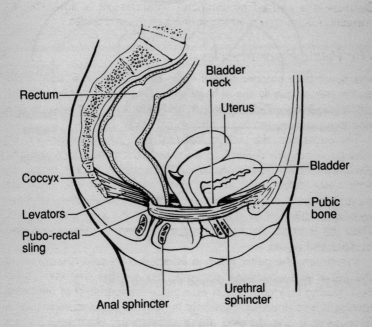

Figure 1: Side view of the female pelvic floor and pelvic organs

In order to get a better idea of where these muscles are in your body, look at figure 1. The pelvic floor muscles run from the front to the back of the bony pelvis between the pubic bone in front and the coccyx (or tail bone) behind. The urethra, vagina and bowel pass from within the abdominal cavity to the exterior by passing between the pelvic floor muscles which lie on each side. Around the urethra and the anus you can see the sphincter muscles of each lying below the level of the pelvic floor sling. Men should look at figure 7, page 89.

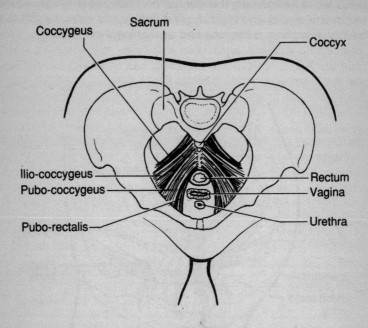

Figure 2: The Pelvic Floor Viewed From Above

Now look at figure 2. In this view of the muscles you can appreciate how the pelvic floor muscles fill in the gap between the bones of the true pelvis, supporting the internal organs. The muscles form a broad V-shaped gutter spanning the pelvic cavity from side to side as well as from front to back. These muscles are collectively known as the **levators** and are made up of various parts – coccygeus (pronounced coxi-jee-us), ilio-coccygeus and pubo-coccygeus. Part of the pubo-coccygeus muscle loops around the lower part of the rectum and is called the pubo-rectal sling. Notice that the levator muscles lie on either side of the rectum, vagina and urethra and do not constrict them. The levators are mainly muscles of support.

Viewed from below, as in figure 3, the levators are again seen to be placed at a distance from the urethra. They are deeply placed muscles. Just beneath the skin of the perineal area are weaker, superficial muscles which surround the vaginal opening and have sexual functions, being attached at the front to the clitoris. These muscles have only a weak effect in helping to control the bladder and urethra. It is clear that the major part of urinary control relies on the urethral sphincter muscles themselves.

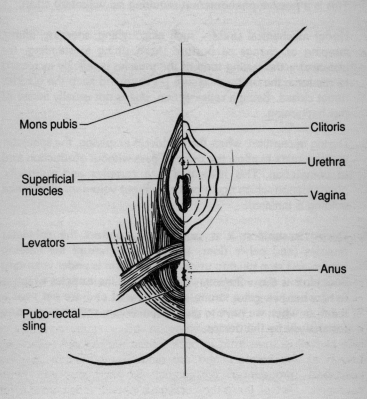

Figure 3: **The pelvic floor viewed from below**

Mons pubis
Clitoris
Urethra
Superficial muscles
Vagina
Levators
Anus
Pubo-rectal sling

The Urethral Sphincter Muscles

The sphincter muscles are wrapped closely around the urethra to act as a control valve. They have several functions:

1. At rest, they maintain a constant tone which exerts pressure on the urethra, keeping it closed – the urethral closure pressure. This is a passive phenomenon requiring no voluntary effort.

2. Under mechanical stress – such as coughing, sneezing, lifting, jumping or change of posture (from sitting to standing, for instance) – the resting tone of the muscles is reflexly increased to reinforce the urethral closure pressure and keep the bladder outlet closed. Being a reflex action, one is not usually aware of this happening.

3. During micturition, when the bladder is emptying, the sphincter muscles relax to allow the urine to pass without obstruction and to completion. This relaxation is a complex and automatic phenomenon which again occurs without voluntary effort once voiding is initiated.

4. During micturition it is possible to contract the sphincter muscles (and pelvic floor) in order to interrupt the voiding stream and stop passing urine. This function is under voluntary control. It is this voluntary contraction of the muscles which is used when we get a strong desire to void and are not near a toilet, or when we have to give a mid-stream specimen of urine for analysis by the doctor.

The Causes of Incontinence – Effects of Sphincter Weakness

Weakness of the urethral sphincter muscles can affect all or some of these normal functions. The first sign of weakness is usually seen under conditions of mechanical stress when the intra-abdominal pressure is raised by coughing, sneezing, straining or lifting. If the muscles fail to increase the urethral closure pressure sufficiently, urine will leak out at the time of the stress. This is called **stress incontinence.** It can occur with simple events such as a single cough or sneeze, or only with more severe provocation such as getting out of a chair, running or lifting. Some people only experience leakage under conditions of extreme stress such as aerobic exercises, tennis or skipping and trampoline-type exercises.

When the muscles are severely damaged and weakened, the passive tone may be diminished. Leakage of urine may then occur without obvious stress or provocation, resulting in **dribble incontinence.** This type of leakage can also occur if the bladder is chronically overdistended due to failure to empty completely. The condition is then referred to as **overflow incontinence.**

If the voluntary closure mechanism is deficient it will be impossible to stop the urinary stream during micturition. On testing, it was found that about 30% of women cannot interrupt the voiding stream. In the elderly up to 50% cannot do so. Not all of these women are incontinent because generally most people stay dry by automatic and involuntary control of the bladder and sphincter muscles.

Voluntary control is important, however, when we get a strong desire to pass urine and are not near a toilet. This urgent desire to void is due to overactive contractions of the bladder itself – a condition called the **unstable bladder.** If urine leaks out at the time of the unstable bladder contractions before a toilet can be reached, it is called **urge incontinence.** Sometimes the whole bladder contents can be lost under these circumstances, resulting in **flooding incontinence.** It is this type of problem which affects adolescent girls who leak when they are laughing or giggling and cannot control the flow.

Another way in which the unstable bladder can manifest itself is by causing **bedwetting.** In this condition the bladder contracts to empty during episodes of deep sleep such that the sufferer is usually not woken by the wetting episode. In adults it is unusual to have persistent bedwetting without also having a bladder control problem (usually urge incontinence) by day. Urge incontinence itself grows more common and more severe with advancing years and is extremely troublesome in the elderly. If you have this type of problem you will also need to read the section on bladder training.

The strength and competence of the urethral sphincter muscles is thus an important factor in many different types of urinary incontinence. Because some parts of the sphincter muscles have the same derivation as the levator muscles they have similar nerve supplies. Thus exercise of one group of muscles generally exercises all. Although it is possible to learn differential control of these muscles, enabling one to pass urine (by relaxation of the urethral sphincter) whilst retaining bowel gas (by contraction of the anal sphincter), few individuals actually succeed in doing so. Thus the sphincter muscles generally move and contract in conjunction with the large pelvic floor muscles and the best way to improve them is by a programme of 'pelvic floor exercises'. These exercises are designed to strengthen and tone up the muscles around the urethra and pelvic floor and are a vital part of regaining urinary control.

The exercise programme which follows warrants your careful attention and regular practice. Even with exercise, all muscles take time to strengthen so do not be impatient. After all, Mr Universe didn't get his bulging biceps in 5 minutes. It often takes 6 to 10 weeks to really get enough strength back into the muscles for improvement to show. Don't get discouraged if progress is slow, especially if you have had many children or are elderly or obese.

If you are overweight your chances of success on this programme will be diminished. Therefore, a few words about weight control are in order.

Weight Control

Excess weight is an unnecessary burden on a weak pelvic floor. In addition, it is a burden which you carry around with you all the time. Consequently, the pelvic floor muscles are constantly being stretched and weakened. This makes pelvic floor exercises both difficult to perform and less effective and thus significantly delays progress.

If you are serious about wanting to regain bladder control you **must** shed those excess kilos. Crash diets are not recommended. The excess weight went on slowly in most people, often over a number of years, and it is best to take it off slowly. It really doesn't matter which weight-reduction diet you choose to follow provided you stick to it. If there is something in the diet regimen you have chosen which you do not like eating, **do not** substitute something which you do like eating. Simply go without. Remember, you are trying to lose weight and the more you eat the longer it is going to take. Try to select a dietary regimen that you can stick to without great hardship and then discipline yourself to follow it.

Avoid repeated short-lived starvation dieting followed by a return to normal food intake which causes the weight to return. The body soon gets used to this 'feast and famine' rotation and responds by subtle changes in the way it regulates its fat stores. As a consequence it becomes progressively more difficult to lose weight with the next diet, and much easier to put the weight back on when you give up your diet in disgust!

Most overweight people deny eating excessively. That is not the point. The fact is that every overweight person eats more than their body requires otherwise they would not be overweight. If you are carrying excess weight you must learn to eat less all the time. In other words, you must change your eating habits forever.

Check your weight only once a week, either wearing the same clothing or without any. Record your weight in kilogrammes each week. Aim to lose 0.5 to 1kg (1 to 2 pounds) **every** week. We are looking for slow, progressive and sustained weight loss. If the weight does not come off, eat even less. Do not have a celebratory 'binge', and, above all, don't cheat. You will feel much better generally for getting into good shape and your exercise programme will be more likely to be effective. There are some basic rules to be followed if you are to be successful:

- Eat at regular meal times only. Don't skip lunch.
- Eat only at the dining table. Don't 'snack' between meals.
- Eat slowly and enjoy your food.
- Eat small portions.
- Eat sensibly.
- Avoid alcohol and all fatty foods.
- Always do your food shopping on a full stomach and buy only what is on your list.
- Don't overstock the house with food.
- Choose high-fibre foods.
- Don't think of yourself as dieting — you're eating sensibly, forever.

General Health Considerations

Many factors may aggravate a bladder control problem and some of these may require attention during the course of your exercise programme if you are to be successful. Weight reduction has already been mentioned and is extremely important. Constipation, anxiety, urinary infections, general health and posture can all have adverse effects upon the bladder.

Constipation

Constipation is common in our society as a result of our increasingly sedentary way of life and refined dietary habits. A loaded bowel may press on the bladder, but most of the damage is done during attempts to empty the constipated colon by straining. Straining down to have the bowel opened can undo all the hard work you have put in during your pelvic floor exercises. Straining stretches the pelvic floor muscles and weakens them again.

If you suffer from constipation, you need to change your diet to include more roughage and fibre. Fresh fruit and vegetables are helpful in this regard, but you will also need to increase your fibre intake with bran and high-fibre breads. Bran can be obtained either as unprocessed bran, which is cheap but not very palatable, or as bran-containing breakfast cereals. Bran is a natural laxative because of the fibre it contains. It is not absorbed by the body and therefore retains water in the motion, making it softer and easier to pass. It also has important additional benefits in reducing the incidence of gall stones and diverticular disease, both of which are common in middle aged and elderly women. For it to be effective, you must take enough bran. With unprocessed bran, 3 heaped tablespoons or more per day may be necessary. Sprinkle it on other cereals or fruit, and use it to thicken soups or gravy to disguise it. Start by adding one teaspoonful of bran a day and increasing the amount by one teaspoonful every three to four days. When you are taking enough regularly, the motions will be softer and bulkier and straining will no longer be required. If too much bran is taken it will produce abdominal pain and large amounts of bowel gas — in some instances even bowel incontinence.

Do not use laxatives and purgatives unless it is essential. Remember that it is not necessary for the bowels to open every day for you to stay healthy. Constipation means that the motions are hard and difficult to pass. Regular use of laxatives on the erroneous assumption that the bowel must be opened every morning is both harmful and unnecessary. Consult your family doctor if natural dietary remedies and attention to fluid intake do not have the desired effect or if your bowel habit changes suddenly without cause. Also report blood in the motion. **Don't strain.**

Chronic coughing

A chronic cough is usually caused by excessive smoking or lung disease. If you are a smoker, cut down. Take shorter puffs on your cigarette and inhale less of the smoke. Take a greater time between puffs. Throw away larger butts. Give up entirely if you can.

If you have other lung disease seek advice from your family doctor about more effective treatment or ask about chest physiotherapy. Hay fever sufferers should consider desensitization programmes which are available through most hospitals.

Anxiety

Emotional stress and anxiety can severely affect bladder control. If you have problems in this area you may need professional help in overcoming them. Stress management courses are widely available and are advertised in the daily newspapers. Specialized courses are run by many colleges and by some private psychologists. Relaxation exercises can be learned and can help most people to overcome their anxiety problems. In some cases, individual counselling may be required to identify and rectify the cause of the problem.

The first step in this process is the realization that you have an anxiety problem and that it can affect your bladder. The next step is to seek some help. This is not an admission of failure on your part, nor is it something to be ashamed about. Take courage and talk to your doctor or district nurse about your worries and take their advice. Many problems in our lives are diminished by sharing them with others. Just unburdening yourself may improve the way you feel about life and help you to cope.

Drugs

Some drugs can affect the way your bladder works and reduce the effectiveness of the pelvic floor and sphincter muscles. Tablets taken for blood pressure control are particularly prone to do this. Prazosin (Hypovase) and phenoxybenzamine (Dibenyline) have been known to cause incontinence. Such drugs should only be stopped or changed after full consultation with your doctor. Diuretics (water pills) can be extremely troublesome, especially if they are fast acting 'loop' diuretics. Talk to your doctor about changing to a slower-acting diuretic if you are taking one of these agents. Many drugs taken for pain and arthritis cause constipation. Sleeping tablets may cause night incontinence. If you are taking *any* drugs, check with your doctor that they do not have known side-effects on bladder, bowel or pelvic floor and sphincter muscles. Note that coffee and tea, because of the caffeine that they contain, can also act as diuretic agents (see advice in the section on fluid intake). Alcohol can have similar effects.

Diabetes

Diabetes mellitus can affect the nerve supply to the bladder and urethra. Happily this is rare and most diabetics will respond to this and similar exercise programmes provided that they reduce weight, maintain good diabetic control and do the exercises. Diabetics are more prone to urinary infections than other people and this needs to be checked.

Urinary Infections

Cystitis and associated inflammation of the bladder and urethra can adversely affect bladder control. The symptoms are frequent passage of small amounts of urine due to bladder discomfort and irritation both day and night, and burning or stinging sensations on passing urine. The urine may smell 'fishy' and sometimes becomes cloudy or blood-stained. Some people get fever and loin pain. Early treatment is required.

If you think you have a urinary infection, start to drink even more – 3 litres (5¼ pints) a day. See your family doctor as soon as possible and get him to arrange a urine culture and to start you on a course of antibiotics. Take the entire course of antibiotics as directed even if the symptoms abate within a day or two. Proprietary remedies available over the counter from your local chemist can alleviate the discomfort of cystitis. If symptoms persist, consult your doctor again for another urine culture.

Sometimes recurrent infections are related to intercourse or poor hygiene. There are some simple measures you can take to reduce the risk:

Keep the genital area clean — shower regularly but also take a bath at least once a week.

Drink plenty of liquid – aim to keep the urine dilute.

Make sure you empty the bladder completely every time you void.

Always wipe yourself from front to back, **not** back to front.

Remember to empty the bladder after intercourse.

Wear only cotton underwear and tights with a cotton gusset.

If you are troubled by recurrent infections or repeated attacks of 'cystitis' symptoms despite these precautions you will need further investigation. There may be something minor causing the problem, such as low-grade bladder inflammation, or there may be something more serious. Never ignore blood in the urine – it is never normal and may indicate underlying disease such as stones or tumours which require early treatment by a specialist.

General Posture

A good posture when standing or sitting will improve more than your morale and appearance. Slouching about with round shoulders and stomach bulging not only makes you look and feel prematurely old but puts additional strain on the pelvic floor and back muscles. Get into the habit of standing tall. Use your abdominal or tummy muscles to control your protruding stomach. Watch those drooping shoulders and straighten up your back. Check your position in a mirror. Half the problem is just not caring what you look like. As you regain your bladder control you will want to get out more and start joining in life once again. Start to take a pride in your appearance right now. Improving your posture will make you feel more alive and take strain off your back and pelvic floor. Keep watching your weight.

Personal Hygiene

Many incontinent people have a strong fear of being 'smelly' even if they leak only infrequently and small amounts. This is understandable but you should guard against becoming irrational about this. Simple hygienic measures will prevent odour becoming a problem.

Keep the genital area clean and dry. Shower regularly but avoid over-zealous washing and highly scented soaps. Take a bath once or twice a week and let the water enter the vagina to remove any discharge. There is no need to use disinfectant solutions — a simple soap is perfectly adequate. Always dry the area thoroughly by patting rather than vigorously rubbing, which can irritate the skin.

If incontinence is sufficiently severe to cause constant wetness of the skin and soreness try a rinsing with cool water each time you empty the bladder and dry the genital area off with a hair dryer. Try changing to glycerine soap unperfumed, or simple, pure baby soap for a while.

Avoid excessive sweating and dampness. Wet skin is prone to fungal infections and ulceration. Choose only pure cotton underwear which is not too tight. If you wear tights, ensure they have a cotton gusset; in summer switch to stockings or go without. Change underwear regularly. If you are wearing a protective pad change it soon after it becomes damp. Try to select loose, airy clothing, especially in summer. If necessary use a simple talc or dusting powder. Discard all nylon underwear and stop using 'step-ins', 'roll-ons' or other elasticated garments.

Keep the urine dilute by keeping up your fluid intake. Aim to keep the urine a pale lemon yellow colour even in summer. This will reduce the odour of any urine that does leak and the skin irritation that it can cause. If the urine becomes very smelly or burns and stings, suspect an infection and consult your doctor (see above). Skin irritation from urine can be avoided by a silicone barrier cream. If there is severe irritation of the skin or ulceration a 0.5% Boracic acid cream is frequently curative. You can obtain this without prescription from your local pharmacy.

Get vaginal discharges treated promptly. In younger women and diabetics, vaginal infections due to Candida ('Thrush') cause an itchy, white or creamy discharge often after a course of antibiotics for urinary infection. A thinner discharge may indicate Trichomonas infection and a bloody discharge between periods should never be overlooked. After the menopause, vaginal irritation and soreness can result from lack of female hormones and is easily treated by hormone creams. Consult your family doctor promptly as early treatment is important.

Avoid using deodorants, antiseptics and disinfectants in the vaginal area. These substances irritate the sensitive skin in the area and should not be used.

Environmental Factors

Some elements of our everyday environment can affect bladder control. Most people are aware of the effect of cold weather in causing increased frequency of urination and urgency. Little can be done to change this apart from taking more care on such days. However, some factors can be changed and consideration should be given to these if they seem appropriate to your own situation.

Tight clothing or multiple layers of clothing may cause considerable delay between arriving at the toilet and being ready to pass urine. This is especially true if you have to struggle out of slacks, tights and pants before you can sit down. Wear looser clothing which is easier to get out of, especially if you have urge incontinence or are old or disabled. Velcro fasteners on clothing are often easier and quicker to release than zips or buttons.

Low or soft chairs which are difficult to get out of can both delay progress to the toilet and provoke unstable contractions (and urge incontinence) as you rise from them. Try using a firmer or higher chair from which it is easy for you to get up. A chair with solid arms can be helpful to the elderly.

The position of your toilet in the house may have an effect on whether you can reach it in time. This is particularly true for those with arthritis or other disabilities which affect how quickly they can walk. Clearly the toilet cannot be moved in most homes. However, if there is a problem getting to the toilet at night, you should consider getting a commode to put in the bedroom or close by. This is certainly well worth considering if you are caring for an elderly relative with this sort of problem. Take a critical look at the usual pathway to the toilet. Poor lighting, stairs without adequate hand rails, slippery floors or loose rugs are not only dangerous but cause delay in reaching the toilet. Make the necessary corrections if these are appropriate. In addition, make sure that footwear is of a non-slip variety.

Attention to such simple environmental factors can often make a considerable difference to the frequency and severity of the incontinence you experience. While they do not cure the underlying problem, they do make a considerable difference to the quality of life.

Fluid Intake

Many people who suffer from incontinence get into the habit of restricting their fluid intake and going to the toilet frequently, 'just in case'. They do this in the hope of avoiding an accident in public. Unfortunately it is a pernicious habit and over a period of time makes matters considerably worse rather than better. After some time the bladder shrinks because it is never asked to hold very much urine, and eventually it won't hold very much urine. The result is that such people have to visit the toilet more and more frequently by day and find, quite often, that they cannot sleep through the night. This is to be avoided.

The way to prevent this from happening is to stretch the bladder by drinking more and to stop going to the toilet 'just in case'. During your exercise programme, get into the habit of drinking about **2 litres (3½ pints) of fluid a day.** That is approximately 10 to 12 full cups or glasses of liquid each day. What you drink does not matter provided that it isn't fattening. Coffee, tea and other caffeine-containing beverages can affect the bladder of some people. You will have to find out by trial and error whether your bladder is sensitive to caffeine or not. If it is, you should cut down on tea and coffee or try one of the many decaffeinated coffee and tea beverages that are now on the market. Stop going to the toilet 'just in case'.

Be sure to keep your fluid intake up to the 2 litre mark every day. Only go to the toilet when your bladder is full. We recommend that you keep a record of when you go to the toilet and how much urine you pass on a time and volume chart (see page 61). Aim to increase the amount your bladder will hold slowly and progressively week by week. Keeping a written record will encourage you to try harder and you will soon see some progress as you begin to stretch your bladder. It is advisable to space out your fluid intake and avoid drinking more than two cups of fluid at any one session. This ensures that large volumes of urine do not reach the bladder quickly leading to urgency. There is usually no advantage to stopping drinks totally before bedtime. However, it is sensible not to drink large volumes before going to bed if you have a bedwetting problem.

Section Two

Pelvic Floor Exercises

Pelvic Floor Exercises

Pelvic floor exercises are a series of exercise programmes to build up the muscles of the pelvic floor. As these muscles are not visible from the exterior various techniques have to be learned to ensure that you are developing the right muscle groups.

The most important rules to observe in performing pelvic floor exercises are as follows:

1. Do them properly – using and developing the correct muscles.
2. Do them regularly – several times **every** day.
3. Do them intelligently – learning to use the muscles when you most need them.
4. Keep on doing them – nobody stays fit without some exercise.

Keep these rules in mind if you want to make and maintain progress.

About a third of the women who join our programme do not know how to contract the pelvic floor muscles when they start. When asked to do so, they generally respond by 'bearing down' or straining as though to expel a baby. This is a disastrous mistake and actually makes incontinence worse. Others think that pelvic floor contractions involve squeezing the buttocks together, tightening the thigh muscles or pressing the knees together. None of these is a pelvic floor exercise and they will never improve the sphincter muscles which control urine release. At best they may improve the shape of the thighs and buttocks, but that is hardly the point of the exercise.

Remember that the pelvic floor and sphincter muscles are designed to keep your insides inside. The urethral sphincter controls the bladder outlet, the anal sphincter controls the bowel. The pelvic floor levator muscles which pass on either side of the urethra, vagina and rectum, support the pelvic and abdominal organs. Pelvic floor exercises are intended to strengthen all these muscles to restore continence.

It is vital from the outset that you discover which muscles to exercise and for that we recommend that you work through all the following preparatory exercises slowly and deliberately. Make sure that you understand what is required in each of the 'action concepts' and then go and do them.

Preparatory Exercise Programme

This section is designed to get you to start using the correct muscles. As you read, do the appropriate action and concentrate on the outcome. Make sure you do **all** these preparatory exercises before proceeding further. Tick them off on the record of progress (page 51) as you do them.

Exercise 1.

Imagine trying to stop yourself from passing wind from the bowel. Surely you have had to do that at some time in the past? To control the wind you must contract the anal sphincter muscle surrounding the back passage. As you read, try contracting that muscle as if you really did have wind. Do it now. You should be able to feel the muscle move. The buttocks and thighs should not move at all. You should be aware of the skin around the anus contracting and the anus being pulled upwards away from whatever you are sitting on. Really concentrate on experiencing this.

Exercise 2.

Now imagine that you are sitting on the toilet passing urine. Envisage trying to stop the flow of the urine. Really try to stop it. Try doing that now as you are reading. You should be using the same group of muscles, but whereas you may easily be able to control the bowel gas, controlling the flow of urine is more difficult because of the higher pressures which the bladder can generate. Next time you go to the toilet to pass urine try this 'stop test' about half way through emptying your bladder. Once you have stopped the flow, relax again and allow the bladder to empty completely. Possibly you will only be able to slow down the stream because your muscles are weak. Don't worry, they will improve in time. If the stream speeds up when you try this exercise, you are contracting the wrong muscles. **Do not** get into the habit of doing the 'stop test' every time you pass urine. This exercise should be performed **only once a day at maximum**.

Exercise 3.

Next imagine lying on your back on a bed with your legs bent and knees wide apart. Envisage someone trying to stick a pin into you in the perineal area between the vagina and anus (or just in front of the anus if you are male). Without moving your legs or holding your breath, and keeping your bottom fixed on the bed, try to pull your perineum back inside your body and away from the pin by contracting the pelvic floor muscles. Really see that pin in your mind's eye and pull in hard. Try this for yourself in practice next time you get the opportunity. At first there will not be much movement away from the pin, but if you watch what happens with a mirror, you will see some movement and notice the anal skin corrugating and moving forwards. Put your finger on the perineum and feel it move as you contract the muscles. Concentrate and work hard. When you relax again feel the perineum fall back onto your finger.

Exercise 4.

In the same position, put a finger of one hand on the tail bone (the coccyx) which you will feel just behind the anus. Put a finger of the other hand on the pubic bone which you will feel in the pubic hair above the clitoris (or the penis in the male). By contracting the pelvic floor muscles try to bring your two fingers closer together. You should feel a slight movement of the tail bone up towards the pubic bone as you contract the muscles. The pelvic floor muscles are modified from muscles which wag the tail of lower species of animals. In the human the coccyx is all that remains of the tail. Try wagging up and down what remains of your tail now. Be sure to keep your legs bent and knees apart so that you cannot cheat by using other muscles. Remember the feeling of tension in the pelvic floor muscles in this exercise should be similar to that which you experienced in the previous exercises.

Exercise 5.

This exercise is the most important for women to do. Again, lying on your back with legs bent and knees apart, lubricate the index and middle fingers of your right hand with a cream, lotion or surgical lubricant such as K-Y Jelly. Gently insert first one, then both fingers right inside the vagina. Don't be afraid; this will not harm you. Now separate the fingers as in a 'scissors action', from top to bottom, not from side to side. With the fingers held apart within the vagina, contract the pelvic floor muscles to try to squeeze the fingers together. You will feel most of the action at the back as the pubo-coccygeus and pubo-rectal portions of the levators contract. At first there may be very little movement, especially if you have had large babies or many children or are elderly. If you feel nothing at all it is because you are not trying or not sending the right messages to the muscles. Concentrate and squeeze hard. The muscles are there and you just have to learn how to use them again. Feel not only the movement but the sensation actually in the pelvic floor muscles as you tense them. Notice how slack the muscles are when you relax again. This exercise is crucial to the programme and **must not** be omitted. It will be referred to as **vaginal digital self-assessment.** You may prefer to do this in a warm bath.

Exercise 6.

Now try inserting a tampon into the vagina. Pulling gently on the string, contract the muscles around the vagina trying to retain the tampon within the vagina. If your muscles are very lax you may need to dampen the tampon before insertion and then allow it to swell a little before commencing this exercise.

Men should concentrate on exercises 1 to 4. Remember not to hold your breath or shrug your shoulders during these exercises. The buttock and thigh muscles should also remain relaxed. Some physiotherapists recommend that men try to 'wag' or elevate the penis. Although this can be fun, it does not necessarily involve pelvic floor and sphincter contractions and is not therefore very helpful. It is the perineum which should move and you must concentrate on using the correct muscles of bladder control before going further.

By now you should have a clear idea of which muscles to contract. You will appreciate that all the above exercises require contractions of the same group of muscles. The pelvic floor muscles and sphincter muscles work together in these exercises, closing the urethra and anus and constricting the vagina. Concentrate when you do these exercises. Remember which muscles you are using and the sensation you experience when you contract them.

Having discovered which muscles to exercise, the next step is to commence a programme of regular exercises. It is important, however, to check that you are doing the correct exercises regularly through the programme by vaginal digital self-assessment as described above. Record having done so on your progress chart (page 51).

The Basic Exercise Programme

Basic considerations

Having identified the correct muscles to use in your preparatory exercise programme, 2 further points need to be made before you commence. Firstly, there are 2 types of pelvic floor contractions which you need to practise – **fast** and **slow.**

Fast contractions should be performed in time as you say aloud:

Contract – Relax, Contract – Relax, Contract – Relax...

Make sure that each contraction you do is a **worthwhile contraction**, not just a little twitch of the muscle.

Slow contractions are sustained for between 3 and 4 seconds in time with a slow chant of:

Contract – Two – Three – Four – Relax, Pause, Contract – Two – Three – Four – Relax, Pause, Contract – Two – Three – Four – Relax...

Equal numbers of fast and slow contractions should be performed in any one session of exercises. Practise doing that now, doing 5 fast and 5 slow contractions. Practise doing the same thing whilst lying down in bed (with legs bent and knees apart); sitting on a chair with knees apart; kneeling on all fours, standing and squatting. Make sure that you can **feel** the muscles contracting no matter what your position.

The second point to be aware of at this stage is that it is unrealistic to expect too much of the muscles in the early stages. The pelvic floor and sphincter muscles, being weak and unaccustomed to exercise, tend to get tired easily. This fatigue occurs in all muscles which are being used more often than usual and is quite natural. The importance of this phenomenon lies in the fact that once the sphincter muscles are exercised to the point of fatigue, they feel and stay weakened for some time. Thus leakage of urine can occur more easily during this recovery period. It is important, therefore, to find out, by trial and error, how many contractions **you** can do before the muscles feel tired and their force of contraction begins to weaken.

Determine for yourself now the number of slow contractions you can do before the muscles feel tired. Using vaginal digital self-assessment check the number of contractions again, making sure that each contraction can be felt squeezing your fingers. At first you may find that you can only perform 3, 4, or 5 slow contractions before the muscles feel tired and weak. Others may be able to do more. The important thing at this stage is to establish your own personal number, whatever it is. Record this number in the contractions/session row under Week 1 on your progress chart (figure 4, page 51).

Each exercise session should consist of equal numbers of fast and slow contractions. So if your number of contractions is, say, 4, each session will consist of 4 slow and 4 fast contractions.

Regularity of Exercise

You should start by doing a pelvic floor exercise session, of equal numbers of fast and slow contractions, **10 times** each and every day. If your personal number of contractions is 4 (as above), this will ensure that the muscles contract at least 80 times a day – 4 fast, 4 slow X 10 = 80. Obviously if your number is higher than this you will be doing more contractions each day, but you must do the exercises **ten times** a day, **every** day, to start off with.

Each week you should plan to increase your number of contractions in each session by one or two, depending on progress. Take it slowly and don't overdo it in the early stages. Do, however, make sure that you keep advancing the number of contractions, no matter how slowly, week by week. By the end of the first month you should be doing 200 contractions each day, no matter where you started. Go on pushing yourself to do better than this as time goes by. Record your progress at the end of each week.

This may sound impossible when you first start but you will soon find it easy if you keep practising. You may be wondering how you are going to find the time to do all these exercises, and where to do them. It takes almost no time to perform a single session of pelvic floor exercises because you can do them while you are doing other things. As to where to do them, the answer is anywhere and everywhere.

As a suggestion, try doing an exercise session in each of the following situations.

1. Before getting out of bed
2. Cleaning your teeth
3. Taking a shower
4. Washing up dishes
5. Morning and afternoon tea-break
6. While cooking
7. Waiting at traffic lights or bus-stops
8. After meals
9. Watching television
10. Before going to sleep.

The problem is not when or where to do the exercises but rather **remembering** to do them regularly every day.

Remembering to Exercise

As an aid to memory we recommend that you buy some self-adhesive stickers from a stationers and stick them in places where they will remind you to do your exercises. We suggest places such as the bathroom mirror, shower, over the kitchen sink, cooking stove, refrigerator door, on the TV set, car windscreen, sewing basket and in the laundry. Keep reminding yourself that you are in training. Do a session of exercises every time you see one of your stickers.

Explain to your family what you are doing and enlist their support. Get them to remind you to do the exercises and to encourage you. If you have a close friend get them to take an interest. You need all the support and encouragement you can get.

If you don't do the exercises you will not get better.

Making Progress

As you begin to make progress, increase not only the number of contractions in each session, but also the number of sessions each day. Push yourself to do a little better each day. Support from your family at this time is helpful in maintaining your motivation. The week-by-week programme outline (page 44) will give you a guide to the rate of progress to aim for.

After 6 to 8 weeks you should be doing between 300 and 400

contractions each day and they will start getting easier. When you do contract the muscles, make sure that it is a **worthwhile** contraction. Don't cheat; it doesn't help. **Don't give up.**

Do keep a record of your exercises as this will encourage you to keep up your efforts. Record the number of contractions and number of sessions you have got to at the end of each week. Check your ability to slow or stop the urinary stream in the 'stop test'. Note your average daily fluid intake in cups or glasses of liquid (see section on fluid intake, page 20) and keep a record of how often you pass urine and how much your bladder will hold. The normal bladder will hold 400 to 500ml.

Checking your Progress

As you increase the number and strength of the contractions you will notice an improvement in your ability to slow down or stop the flow of urine when you micturate. Do this 'stop test' only once or twice a week to check on your progress. Do not get disheartened if you cannot stop the flow, everything takes time. Do not get into the habit of stop-start micturition every time you pass your urine. This is a highly dangerous habit because your bladder may respond by becoming unstable (making you even wetter), or by not emptying properly resulting in a risk of recurrent urinary infections. To avoid this problem, get into the habit of **relaxing** when you pass urine. Give yourself time to empty the bladder completely every time. Do not strain to pass urine or to finish off – just relax.

You will also begin to feel an improvement in the strength of the contractions you can feel when you put your fingers in the vagina. You should make this digital vaginal check on your muscle action regularly – 2 or 3 times each week. It will ensure that you are continuing to use the correct muscles, and as you feel the improvement in the strength of the muscles, it will encourage you to try even harder. Digital vaginal assessment of this kind is imperative. It won't do you harm, it isn't dirty or unhygienic, and it doesn't make you go blind. So do it.

Stress-specific Exercises – Using the Muscles Intelligently

Improving the strength and tone of the pelvic floor and sphincter muscles is only one aspect of helping yourself to overcome your incontinence problem. Equally important is the intelligent use of these developing muscles.

For stress incontinence

The pelvic floor and sphincter muscles reflexly contract when you cough or sneeze because that is the way we are all designed. If you leak under such conditions it is because the strength of the reflex activity in the weakened muscles is insufficient to keep the urethra closed. However, you can learn to improve the urethral closure pressure voluntarily during such events by deliberate contraction of the sphincter and pelvic floor muscles. You do have to make a deliberate effort to do this, and the programme below of stress-specific exercises is designed to help you with this.

Try this programme only **after** you have started to make progress with the basic exercise programme and after you are sure that the muscles are improving on vaginal digital self-assessment. If you start too soon you may be disappointed and give up. Generally we recommend that you start these exercises only after 4 to 6 weeks of regular basic exercises. The stress-specific exercises should be performed **in addition** to your on-going basic exercise programme, not as a substitute.

To begin with let us assume that your leakage problem occurs with coughing. This implies that when you cough the reflex activity in the muscles is not sufficiently strong to retain the urine in the bladder. So you must learn to deliberately and voluntarily contract the muscles when you cough in order to augment the urethral closure pressure to keep yourself dry.

Practise doing this exercise with an empty bladder:
    Contract – Cough – Relax, Pause, Contract – Cough – Relax ...
After a few days try:
    Contract – Cough – Cough – Relax, Pause, Contract – Cough – Cough – Relax...

Slowly increase the number of coughs you do up to 5 or 6 whilst keeping up the contraction of the pelvic floor and sphincter muscles. After a week or so, start doing the exercise at increasing intervals of time after you have emptied your bladder. This will ensure that you learn to keep in control when coughing when your bladder is one-third, one-half or three-quarters full.

At first, when practising with more urine in the bladder, just do the contract – cough – relax routine. Slowly work your way up so that you can cough 5 or 6 times even with a full bladder and still stay dry. During this period you should do the exercise whilst sitting, standing and walking. Get into the habit of contracting the muscles every time you feel a cough coming on, and maintain the contraction until it is safe to relax.

What starts off as a deliberate exercise will slowly become second nature to you – like learning to write or ride a bicycle or any of the other complex things we learn to do with great effort and which we now take for granted. This will only happen with practice, practice and more practice.

It is important to remember that in everyday life, your success in achieving control will depend upon your ability to rapidly contract the pelvic floor and sphincter muscles when you feel a cough coming on, and then to sustain the contraction until the danger period is over. That is why you need to practise both the fast and slow contractions in the basic exercise programme. Of course, once you can do this, you have cured your problem.

If you leak under other circumstances you will need to attack these problems in the same manner. Once you are making some progress with the contract – cough – relax exercises, you can advance to other exercises to cover the other situations which cause you to leak. Start off in the same way with each situation that gives you a problem. For example:

Contract – jump – relax
Contract – sneeze – relax
Contract – lift – relax
Contract – skip – relax
Contract – change posture – relax.

Gradually increase the number of jumps, skips, lifts or sneezes you can do with the pelvic floor muscles still contracted. Then slowly increase the amount of fluid in your bladder at the time you do the exercise. Take it slowly and do not try to do too many different things at the same time. If you do have an accident during this time don't get disheartened. Go back in your exercise programme to what you were able to do 3 days previously and confirm that you can still do it. This will build up your self-confidence again. Do the same thing a few times until you feel sure of yourself and when you feel ready for it try the exercise that caused the accident once more. Keep challenging yourself to try harder and do a little better.

For urge incontinence

Pelvic floor contractions are what you almost instinctively do to prevent urinary leakage when you get an urgent desire to void. If you frequently get urgency of this kind you probably have an unstable bladder (see page 55) and you should read the section on bladder training.

In the presence of an unstable bladder contraction giving rise to urgency, pelvic floor contraction has several effects. Firstly, it elevates the base of the bladder and closes the sphincter muscles around the urethra and anus. It is the closure of the urethral sphincter muscles that prevents urine leakage during unstable contractions (or not as the case may be). Secondly, the contraction of the pelvic floor and sphincter muscles suppresses the bladder contraction by a reflex in the spinal cord. This happens more quickly if the pelvic floor contraction is vigorously applied very early on in the course of an unstable bladder contraction before very high pressures are reached. The reflex inhibition of the bladder contraction is also better if the urine never flows and if the 'brake' can be applied with persistence. Obviously if the pelvic floor and sphincter muscles are relaxed before the bladder contraction has gone away, leakage will occur. With practice you will find that the muscles get stronger and you will find that the bladder contractions do go away if they meet sufficiently determined resistance. Once the bladder contraction has been suppressed in this way there is no longer any danger of leakage on the way to the toilet. Indeed, at a later stage, you will find that it may be 20 or 30 minutes before you get another desire to void.

Period Time

Be careful at period time. The hormonal changes which accompany menstruation can affect the pelvic muscles and you may find that you are not as good at this time as you were previously. Don't let this undermine your confidence and determination. Keep practising. By the time of your next period you may have made more progress and you will be able to feel justifiably proud of yourself.

Try not to fall into the trap of giving up your exercise programme during the days you are menstruating. The muscles still work at this time and there is no excuse at all for not trying. Too often people tell themselves that they can't do something at period time because they won't even make the effort. Tell yourself that you **can** do it and in time you **will** do it.

Building up Your Self-confidence

Pads and incontinence appliances have an important part to play in the lives of people with incontinence. They enable sufferers to cope with the problem and go on living a full and rewarding life. Many people use them as 'safety nets' for use especially when going out of the house or playing sport. In the early stages of your exercise programme this is a wise precaution to take. Unfortunately you can come to rely upon these devices too much.

After 4 to 6 weeks on the programme and once you have started the stress-specific exercises and noticed some improvement in your control and self-confidence, try leaving your pads at home. This will encourage you to try harder and to place more reliance upon your own muscles. Once you are successful celebrate by buying yourself a new piece of clothing or some new underwear. What you save from not buying pads that you no longer need will soon pay for the extravagance, and you will feel a lot better for it.

Remember the warning about difficulties that some women experience at the time of the menstrual period. Some women have trouble in the week prior to the period, others do so during the period itself and for a day or so afterwards. Others have no trouble at all. Be prepared if you are one of the unfortunate ones. As you progress you may find that you are able to stay dry and in control by using a tampon. A tampon in the vagina gives added support to the urethra and augments your muscular control even on bad days. Change the tampon at least every 24 hours, otherwise pelvic shock syndrome may occur due to bacteria on the tampon finding their way to the abdominal cavity. Remaining dry in this way is surely preferable to leaking and using a pad to 'mop up' the spillage. Try it and see if it helps you. Whatever happens, don't let a bad few days undermine your self-confidence and stop you from trying. Your determination to succeed is an important factor in overcoming your problem.

If after 8 weeks you are not making progress on your own, consider seeking help. Look at your exercise record chart. If it is mainly blank, you probably have not been putting in full effort. **Start again.** You can't expect to make progress if you try to take short cuts. However, if you really have been doing your best, this may be the time to seek professional help. The section on adjunctive therapy (page 41) outlines the sort of help that is available.

Pregnancy or Pelvic Operations

A first or further pregancy can be a problem. During the last 3 months of the pregnancy the baby enlarges and presses on the bladder and pelvic floor. At the same time special hormones relax the pelvic floor and pelvic ligaments preparatory to delivery. Up to 42% of women experience stress incontinence at this stage of pregnancy. A great many of them will continue to have leakage after delivery of the baby and although some get better after 3 months, one-third of them will have persistent incontinence for many years.

In order to prevent this, there is a growing tendency for antenatal classes to include a course of pelvic floor exercises. If you had a bladder control problem before the pregnancy or during a previous pregnancy, a further course of intensive pelvic floor exercises is essential for you. You should start early in the pregnancy and continue throughout and for at least 3 months after delivery. A great many women could avoid troublesome and persistent bladder control problems associated with pregnancy and childbirth by taking the trouble to do pelvic floor exercises conscientiously. Prevention is better than cure.

After the birth of the baby, you must recommence your pelvic floor exercises as soon as possible. Even if the whole area is sore and numb, the sooner you begin exercising again the better. The longer those stretched, battered and bruised muscles are left without exercise, the longer it will take you to get them working again. Start the day after your delivery – even if you have had a Caesarean section. Keep them up even if it hurts to do so – you won't do any harm. Keep going once you get home and don't give up.

Hysterectomy and other pelvic and lower abdominal operations can be followed by a period of incontinence. If you know that you are to have such an operation, start pelvic floor exercises about 6 weeks before surgery and recommence them the day after the operation. It may be sore and difficult but be determined. You will do no harm and may save yourself a good deal of subsequent trouble and anguish.

Improving Your Sex Life

Once you begin to feel some improvement in the pelvic floor muscles during your regular digital vaginal self-assessment, you are ready to start making some improvements in your sex life. This is a pleasant additional benefit from your pelvic floor exercise programme. You must be able to feel with your fingers the contractions of the pelvic muscles before you are ready to surprise your sexual partner.

During intercourse try contracting your pelvic floor muscles. This is clearly best done in quiet moments rather than during vigorous thrusting. Start in the woman-below position and try a few fast and a few slow contractions. Ask your partner to tell you if he feels anything if he doesn't appear to notice. He should feel your pelvic muscles squeezing the shaft of his penis.

Try the same exercise in the woman-above position where you are in control of the depth and rate of penetration. Try squeezing first the shaft and then the tip of the penis. Encourage your partner to tell you how it feels and whether he prefers slow or fast contractions. Then get him to contract his pelvic floor muscles. This causes the penis to swell and to move. You should be able to feel this movement and swelling within the vagina. Tell him what you feel.

Many women find that this exercise improves the pleasure that both partners get from intercourse. For the man there is increased stimulation and, if the contractions are performed at the time of his climax, he will experience enhancement of the orgasm and ejaculation. Some men learn to control premature ejaculation with these muscles. After ejaculation, pelvic floor contractions will help him to stay in for longer and keep the penis erect for longer. For the woman, pelvic floor contractions during intercourse will increase genital awareness and improve both vaginal and clitoral sensation.

With practice intercourse should become more satisfying and stimulating for both partners and becomes a time of more intimate sharing and communication. You may be surprised how much better the sexual experience is once you begin this active pelvic participation. Above all you should aim to have fun together – it shouldn't be a chore.

Some women have problems with vaginal or bladder irritation, soreness or pain during or after intercourse. This is most commonly due to poor vaginal lubrication either due to lack of arousal or following hysterectomy or after the menopause. This situation is easily overcome by the use of a simple vaginal lubricant such as K-Y jelly, which is freely available at all pharmacies. It is much better to use this type of product than to suffer the agony and apprehension associated with inadequate lubrication. Try to talk to your partner about this, even getting him to put the jelly around the entrance to the vagina for you as a part of fore-play. Both partners are supposed to enjoy intercourse so don't just 'grin and bear it'.

If you have a tendency to get urinary infections or cystitis, remember to empty the bladder after sexual intercourse before going to sleep. This will have the effect of washing out any bacteria that have got into the bladder. Any symptoms of burning or stinging that you may experience the following morning will usually respond to drinking plenty of liquid and do not necessarily warrant antibiotics.

A few women are afflicted by urinary leakage during intercourse. Obviously it is wise for these individuals to empty their bladder beforehand in order to avoid this embarrassing and inhibiting type of leakage. Use of the pelvic floor muscles can sometimes prevent leakage under these circumstances if you are in a position where you have the presence of mind to use them! In a few cases, what leaks out is not urine but a clear, slightly sticky mucous from the glands lining the urethra itself. This is the female equivalent of semen and is nothing to worry about. If true urinary leakage persists don't be too embarrassed to seek professional advice from your doctor before your marriage begins to suffer.

Adjunctive Therapy

If you are having difficulty making progress with your exercise programme, or are unsure that what you are doing is correct, you may benefit from the help of a physiotherapist or specialist training centre. There are several additional measures which are available to help you and these are outlined below. They all involve you seeking help with your problem from someone else. Don't be ashamed, bashful or embarrassed about seeking this help if you need it.

Electrostimulation of the muscles – Interferential therapy

It has been known for a number of years that electrical stimulation of the pelvic floor muscles can help to restore urinary control. Many of the methods of doing this are unpleasant because of the sensations involved, or impractical because of the devices required. Interferential therapy does not suffer from these disadvantages. It is a gentle and effective way of stimulating the muscles without unpleasant sensory effects at the site of the electrodes and is widely available in most physiotherapy departments and in the rooms of many private physiotherapists.

The electrodes are placed beneath the buttocks and in the pubic area in front whilst you lie comfortably on your back. The special type of current which is applied from the machine generates a stimulating electrical field mid-way between the electrodes and within the pelvis itself. Some people feel a pleasant sensation in the vaginal or perineal area. By varying the current, different types of muscles and nerves can be stimulated, and the blood supply to the pelvic organs may be increased. Current 'surges' can be used to stimulate the large pelvic floor muscles as you do your contractions. Each interferential session lasts 20 to 30 minutes and a course of treatment consists of 12 or so sessions. Generally speaking, the more frequently you have the electrostimulation sessions the more benefit you get. It is not until after 6 to 7 sessions that you will feel the benefit.

Some people notice that after electrostimulation they can

achieve more with their own muscles than they could before the session – being able to stop the flow of urine during micturition for example. Others notice an improvement also in their bowel habit. Quite how this treatment works is unknown at the present time, but it does not work by itself. You must do the exercise programme regularly and intelligently between the sessions.

Biofeedback

Biofeedback is a term which is used to describe a treatment process in which you are shown what the muscles are doing when you contract them in order to reinforce the learning process. Digital vaginal assessment is one example of this. You can feel with your fingers the strength of contraction of the muscles and thus ensure that you use the correct muscles. You can also feel the improvement in the muscles as they gain strength and this encourages you to improve even further.

Various other techniques can be used. The 'Perineometer' is an instrument which measures pelvic floor contractions. A balloon device inserted into the vagina or rectum monitors the compression effect of these contractions. By putting a numerical figure on the strength of the muscles progress can be charted week by week, thus encouraging people to make progress. These devices are generally expensive for the individual but may be available through hospital physiotherapy units or from a continence adviser.

Drug Therapy

Several drugs are available that can improve the tone in the urethral sphincter muscles and improve continence. Most of them have some side effects which make them unsuitable for regular or sustained use. Your doctor may, however, decide to use one of these agents to help you to achieve control during the exercise programme whilst the muscles are building up. Even with drug therapy, the exercise programme and stress-specific exercises must be continued. There is simply no substitute for regaining control with your own healthy muscles. Drugs are only used to help you for a short time.

Bladder Training

If you suffer from urge incontinence as well as stress incontinence you may well need special bladder training in addition to pelvic floor exercises. People with this problem have an overactive or unstable bladder which results in frequent and urgent visits to the toilet, often both day and night. If this is your problem, mention it to your doctor. A separate section of this manual outlines a programme of bladder training which is very effective in helping people to regain full bladder control in this situation. However, it is very important that your doctor excludes urinary infection as a cause of the problem before you start. You may also need referral to a urological specialist for special assistance with this type of problem.

Week-by-week Programme Outline

The following pages contain an outline of the entire programme for you to follow week by week. Even if you manage to make progress faster than suggested, do be sure to keep a record of what you are doing and to continue the exercise programme for a full 12 weeks. This is important if you wish to obtain lasting benefit.

Week 1

Practise all the preparatory exercises (page 25) once or twice daily. Tick them off on the progress chart. Make sure that you are using the correct muscles. Find out how many slow contractions you can do before the muscles feel tired and the contractions begin to weaken (page 29). Practise a session of this number of fast and slow contractions in each of the following situations each day:

lying on your back with legs bent and knees apart
sitting on a firm chair with knees apart
kneeling on all fours
squatting
standing with feet apart.

By the end of the week you may, for example, be doing 5 sessions of 5 fast and 5 slow contractions every day. Record .this under week 1 on your progress chart at the end of the week as 10 contractions/session, 5 sessions/day = 50 contractions/day.

Record your weight and the amount you are drinking each day. Don't cheat – it won't help you. Pencil your goals for the next week into the week 2 column.

Week 2

Increase your number of sessions to 10 each day using the suggestions on page 31 to help you to remember to do them. Using vaginal digital self-assessment (page 27) check each day that you are using the correct muscles.

Get your fluid intake up to 2 litres (3½ pints) every day. Don't forget your weight.

By the end of week 2 you should be doing 10 contractions (5 fast and 5 slow) each session and 10 sessions/day = 100 contractions/day. Make a record of what you **have** done and pencil in a higher target for the next week – say 200/day.

Weeks 3 and 4

Make an effort to increase the number of contractions in each session every few days, remembering to do equal numbers of fast and slow contractions. Keep up your fluid intake and continue to eat sensibly. Check 2 or 3 times each week that you are using the correct muscles by vaginal digital assessment. Once or twice a week try a 'stop test' (page 25) to see how good you are.

By the end of week 4 you should be up to 300 contractions/day. Record this on your progress chart and pencil in a higher target for the following week. Really try to reach this target.

Weeks 5 and 6

Keep increasing the number of contractions in each session and the number of sessions you do. Aim for 400 contractions/day. Start to concentrate on slow, sustained contractions, counting up to 7, or even 10, slowly with each sustained contraction.

Commence stress-specific exercises (page 33). Choose only **one thing** to concentrate on for the next 2 weeks – jumps or coughs but not both. Remember to start off with an empty bladder until you can do 5 or 6 coughs or jumps or skips in a row with the pelvic floor contracted all the time. Record how many jumps or coughs you can do on your chart.

Don't forget to watch your weight and to keep up your fluid intake.

If you have an urge incontinence problem start a bladder training programme (section three) at this point. If you are under the supervision of a specialist centre you may be able to start this earlier but do not do so if you are on your own.

Week 7

Keep doing 400 basic contractions each day.

Start to increase the amount in your bladder when you do the stress-specific exercises by doing your practice session at increasing intervals of time after you have emptied your bladder. Keep your record up to date.

Week 8

Keep doing 400 basic contractions per day. Check your muscles using vaginal digital assessment – you should already feel considerable improvement. Try the 'stop test'.

Continue your first stress-specific programme until you can cough or jump 5 to 10 times in a row with even a full bladder without leakage.

Commence a new programme of stress-specific exercises for the next situation which causes a leakage problem. Remember to start off with an empty bladder as in week 5.

Weeks 9 to 12

Keep doing 400 basic contractions per day and keep watching the fluid and food intake.

Continue all your stress-specific exercises until they become second nature to you. Remember to check the muscles regularly by vaginal assessment.

If at this stage you haven't lost the 10kg (22 pounds) or so of weight that you decided to lose at the start of the programme, give your spouse or a charity £25 as a fine for your sloth and weakness of will. If you have lost the weight, buy a new outfit which fits the new, smaller, you.

At the end of week 12 assess your progress. If you have successfully overcome your problem and are cured you may reduce the number of sessions that you do each day. Do not stop doing exercises altogether. Continue to keep your muscles in good shape by regular daily exercise otherwise they will tend to get weak again as you get older.

If the programme has improved your control but you still have an occasional 'accident', keep up your efforts for a few weeks more until you no longer make any progress. You may benefit by consulting a physiotherapist or a continence adviser so that your efforts can be supervised and help given.

If there has been little or no improvement, consider whether you have really tried or not. Look at your record chart. If it is mainly blank you really have no-one to blame but yourself. Don't be lazy – start again and this time **do the whole thing properly.** If, on the other hand, you really did do your best but still have troublesome leakage, get your doctor to refer you to a specialist for further advice. Do not be put off by comments like 'What do you expect at your age?'. You can be helped.

Maintaining Your Progress

The effects of this exercise programme will persist if you keep the muscles you have developed in good shape by on-going practice. Don't waste all your hard work by falling back into old, sloppy habits. Keep watching your weight and posture. Keep your fluid intake up and remember to do some pelvic floor exercises regularly. Once the muscles are in trim you will not have to exercise as hard, but you should not forget about them altogether.

We recommend that you continue to practise your pelvic floor exercises 4 or 5 times a day in order to maintain the progress you have made. Be sure to do both fast and slow contractions when you do an exercise session. Remember to use the muscles intelligently, contracting them before you cough or sneeze. If your problem starts to return, immediately get back on the programme, starting again at the preparatory exercises and working your way through the entire course.

What If ?

If after a three-month course of regularly and properly performed exercises your incontinence persists you may require an operation. Your exercise programme will not have been a waste of time. Firstly, it was worth a try because 70% of people respond to the programme and avoid surgery. Secondly, even if you need surgery, the results are better and the convalescence shorter if your own muscles are in good shape.

Do not fall into the trap of thinking that an operation will absolve you from the necessity of keeping control of the bladder with your own muscles. Most effective incontinence surgery tightens the bladder and urethral supports, leaving the sphincter muscles more capable of maintaining control. But you will still need to use your own muscle control and should start your exercise programme again within a day or two of the operation.

There are about 100 different operations for urinary incontinence, so you will have to be guided by your specialist. No operation is guaranteed to be successful, but some procedures are noticeably less effective than others. A 'vaginal repair' is an operation designed to control significant prolapse, not incontinence, and is to be avoided unless prolapse is your primary complaint. If you do need an operation, it is well to be sure that it is the right one because if it fails to help you the chances of subsequent success are substantially diminished. If in doubt seek another opinion.

If your incontinence problem is associated with frequency and urgency, or inflammatory symptoms such as pain, burning or blood in the urine you should seek referral to a urologist. You may require further investigation by cystoscopy or urodynamic pressure testing before any other surgery is contemplated.

In Summary

This programme of pelvic floor exercises can significantly improve your chances of regaining full control of your bladder. Remember the basic rules:

Do them properly – check regularly to ensure that you are using the correct muscles by digital vaginal self-assessment. Use the 'stop test' only once or twice a week to monitor progress.

Do them regularly – start with sessions 10 times a day, doing equal numbers of fast and slow contractions. Slowly work up the number of contractions that you do in each session and the number of session each day until you are performing 300 to 400 contractions a day.

Do them intelligently – don't overdo it. Learn to use the muscles when you need them most by a programme of stress-specific exercises. Keep on challenging yourself to do a little better day by day.

Do them persistently – don't give up and stay wet, and don't forget to keep your pelvic floor and sphincter muscles in good shape once you have regained urinary continence. Practise, practise, practise.

Watch your weight – and keep on watching that weight. Very few women grow thinner as they get older, but a great many get wetter. So be on your guard against letting your weight creep back on.

Keep your fluid intake up – don't fall back into the habit of going to the toilet 'just in case'.

If you have problems or difficulties with this programme of exercises or fail to understand some part of this manual, please don't be afraid to ask. Your doctor will be able to explain to you anything which does not appear to be clear. The manual is designed to help you to help yourself. If you don't follow the advice it contains and do the exercises regularly and conscientiously, you cannot expect to improve. It is now up to you.

Go to it!

Week Number

	1	2	3	4	5	6	7	8	9	10	11	12
Weight (kg)												
Preparatory exercises												
anus a 1												
penis p 2												
bottom b 3												
...... b 4												
5												
6												
Basic exercise programme												
Contractions/session												
Sessions/day												
Contractions/day												
Leakage												
Record leaks/day												
Stress-specific exercises												
Record number of coughs:												
jumps:												
etc.												

Figure 4: Record of progress chart

Section Three

Bladder Training

The Unstable Bladder

The normal bladder fills and empties 4 or 5 times each day with little voluntary effort or thought on the part of its owner. Most of the time, while the bladder is slowly filling up, there is very little sensation from the bladder. Only when the bladder is nearly full is a desire to void experienced. If micturition is convenient then the bladder is emptied by simply relaxing and thinking about it. Passing urine does not normally require straining or precise muscular control, it is a physiological bodily function which proceeds to completion automatically once it is started. In fact the more one thinks about the act, the more difficult it becomes!

If, however, when the desire to void is experienced, it is not convenient to pass urine, then it is possible to keep the bladder under control by an act of will. In order to achieve this, it is necessary to suppress the tendency of the bladder to contract when it is full, thereby keeping the pressure within the bladder low. This is something which is learned in childhood between the ages of 2 and 4 years. To do so requires an intact central nervous system, a normal bladder and urethra, motivation and training.

Incorrect training as a child or incomplete learning of bladder control results in what everybody knows as a weak bladder. This implies that the owner cannot suppress the bladder and experiences the need to void urgently and frequently, often both day and night. Children with this problem appear to always 'leave it until the last minute'. When, in addition, the child has an abnormally sound sleep pattern, persistent bed-wetting may also be a problem. Adults find that fluids, especially tea, coffee or alcohol, 'just run through' them.

What is happening in fact is that when the bladder is full it contracts to empty. This gives rise to a knee-crossing, eye-watering, urgent desire to void which it is very difficult to control. This **unstable** bladder contraction is probably familiar to everyone from time to time. It commonly occurs after a party when, after a long drive home, the extreme fullness of the bladder makes it difficult to get the key in the front door quickly enough. It then becomes touch and go whether we will get to the toilet in time. When this happens only rarely, it is all part of being human. When the same thing happens 10 or 15 times a day it becomes a real problem, especially when the urgency of the desire exceeds the speed with which the toilet can be reached. In this case leakage of a few drops of urine, or even total flooding, can occur. This type of urinary leakage is called **urge incontinence.**

Urge incontinence is an extremely common complaint and causes considerable inconvenience and embarrassment to its sufferers. The frequency which so often accompanies it becomes a family joke to all but the victim. Nocturia, or the need to pass urine at night, causes broken sleep and consequent tiredness. The incontinence causes a constant fear of public disgrace through odour or wetness, and progressive loss of self-esteem and self-confidence. Depression and anxiety frequently accompany these problems and tend to make matters worse.

The natural consequence of this is that most people who have the problem take evasive action. In the first instance fluid restriction is tried in order to avoid the frequency. Changes of underwear are kept in the handbag in case of accident. 'Just in case' voiding becomes a way of life, the bladder being emptied long before it is near full to avoid being 'caught short' in the supermarket or on the bus. Often daily activities are reorganized around the known availability of public toilets, the sites of which are carefully memorized. Car trips of any distance become a nightmare, with frequent stops for petrol, the tank never being filled in case another toilet stop is required down the road.

The result is that the bladder is never asked to hold very much urine and slowly but surely it gets worse and worse until it simply won't hold very much urine. At this point some people become bladder hermits, becoming more and more frightened to leave the house. At the back of many people's minds is the deep-rooted fear of becoming a smelly, wet old lady or gentleman.

One of the problems with the unstable bladder is that it just doesn't go away. The leakage that it causes seldom responds to the usual operations for incontinence and drug treatment is not always helpful. There is in fact no easy way out of the problem. However, bladder training is effective and can revolutionize the lives of sufferers of urge incontinence, and the troublesome frequency and night time voiding which accompany it. It does require your complete cooperation. If you are not prepared to make this a top priority in your life and comply with the instructions you are probably wasting your time.

Get out of your mind all your old excuses for your bladder problem and determine right now that you are really going to try. Many people with this problem come along with myths about their bladder being small or having weak kidneys. Generally this is rubbish. If you go on believing these sorts of things, or continue to dwell on what you surmise was the cause of the problem, you will stay as you are. Take yourself in hand and start looking forward with a positive attitude, regardless of your age. You don't have to believe in this training programme, you just have to do it.

Follow the instructions carefully. Be prepared to read and re-read the training programme instructions. We recommend that you read the following sections every week or two during the 3 months of the training programme to remind yourself of what to do and how to proceed.

Before You Start

Before you start on a bladder training programme it is **vitally important** that your urine is not infected because urinary infection or cystitis can cause similar symptoms to those of the unstable bladder. If in doubt, go to your doctor and get your urine tested. If the urine is infected you will need a full course of antibiotics followed by another urine culture to ensure that your urine is infection-free before commencing on bladder training. Do not overlook this step.

Note also that the recent onset of urge incontinence in the elderly male may indicate that there is obstruction to the outlet from the bladder by an enlarged prostate gland. Usually this also causes a poor urinary stream, delay or difficulty starting to urinate, dribbling at the end of the stream and sometimes a feeling of incomplete bladder emptying. Any obstruction to the bladder outlet can cause the bladder to become unstable. Usually the bladder settles down again after the obstruction is removed. If in doubt, consult your doctor or a specialist.

In some men the symptoms of frequency, urgency and incontinence persist even after prostate operations. Bladder training can be of considerable benefit under these circumstances.

If your bladder problem is associated with or the result of some disease of the nervous system – such as multiple sclerosis, a stroke, Parkinson's disease or spinal injury – you will probably not be helped by this training programme. Don't lose heart. Your bladder control problem can often be helped by simple medication to calm down your overactive bladder. Go and ask your doctor for help or get referred to a specialist.

For the vast majority of people with an unstable bladder there is no particular cause for the problem. Often it is a 'hang-over' from imperfect training or bedwetting as a child. Commonly it arises slowly over a period of years, gradually getting worse until it becomes intolerable. It is just this situation which the programme was designed to help. Get started!

The Bladder Training Programme

This bladder training programme takes about **3 months** to completely alter your bladder function even though some people get considerable benefit within the first week or two. Your attitude, willingness and determination to succeed are important ingredients in the curative process. Once you have learned how to keep control of your bladder and once again become the master of it, instead of a slave to it, and have practised this skill repeatedly, you will never again have your bladder problem.

The programme is designed to help people with an unstable bladder, but not everyone is the same and not everyone tries as hard. Success on this programme is dependent upon consistent effort on your part. If you will put in 3 months of persistent hard work you will significantly improve the way your bladder works, increasing its capacity, voiding less often and having fewer and fewer 'accidents'.

The programme will also help people with frequency and urgency due to an 'oversensitive' bladder, provided that they do not have urinary infection. Such individuals usually get some discomfort when the bladder is filling up and get into the habit of going frequently to avoid this. In such cases the training programme can desensitize the bladder so that it can hold more without discomfort.

Some people need more help with this programme than others and there are continence clinics in some hospitals and health centres which have been set up to give you assistance. Your own doctor should be able to direct you to one of these if you find that you need help or advice. Don't be afraid to admit that you need help — many people have benefited from the expertise that these clinics have developed.

Your unstable bladder contracts inappropriately in response to filling (often to only low volume) or to provocation (such as change of posture, running water, exercise or intercourse). When it does contract, it pulls open the neck of the bladder, which is normally closed and water-tight, exactly in the way it does when you are going to pass urine. When this happens you naturally try to hold on using the muscles around the urethra — the water pipe which runs from the bladder to the exterior. Whether you leak or not under these circumstances depends on two factors: how strong the muscles are, and how strongly the bladder is contracting. Obviously the duration of that unstable bladder contraction may affect whether control can be maintained or not, as does your motivation to remain dry.

You may be aware already of some of the things which make your bladder worse – cold wet days, winter, running water, anxiety and stress, and period time are often mentioned. Similarly, you may have found some things which help you to control the bladder and get to the toilet in time: crossing the legs, pressure on the perineum (the area between the legs or saddle area). It is important to try to learn more about your bladder and the way it works while you are on this programme. It is especially important for you to quickly find out what you can and cannot do with safety. Once you have determined for yourself your own limits, you can learn how to stay in control of your bladder and slowly improve what you can do.

The aim of the training programme is to increase the capacity of your bladder until it can hold the normal amount of between 400 and 500ml of urine (20 to 25fl oz). In achieving this you need to learn how to suppress your bladder contractions by using various deferment techniques (see page 70) and to practise these over and over again until they become second nature to you. In addition the muscles around the outlet of the bladder and in the floor of pelvis need to be slowly strengthened by exercises. It is, however, important to realize that the art of bladder control lies in learning to control the pressure inside the bladder from the brain rather than by learning to run faster!

Sometimes problems at home or at work can not only make the bladder problem worse, but also make it difficult to concentrate on the programmes below. Be aware of this and seek help, if necessary from your local doctor. Remember that your doctor can only really help if you are completely honest about what the problems are or what is worrying you. Many people have been helped by relaxation exercises which can teach you how to cope with stress and anxiety, as well as helping the bladder. Don't be too frightened to ask for help or too proud to accept it when it is offered.

Getting Started

The Time and Volume Chart

You must keep a daily record of how your bladder works on a time and volume chart (see figs 5,6). On this you should record the volume of urine which you pass in millilitres, the time of day when you do so and the time interval since you last passed urine. Many people find this an irksome task at first, but it is an essential and crucial part of the bladder training programme and must be done if you are to make progress. If you are not prepared to do this, stop at this point and stay wet. Re-examine your motivation.

You will need to purchase a measuring jug calibrated in millilitres capable of holding up to 1 litre (2 pints) of fluid. Keep this in your toilet at home and rinse it each time you use it to measure how much urine you pass. Keep your time and volume chart and a pencil or pen in the same place and write down your volumes and times immediately.

You should also record in an appropriate column whether you have leaked during that interval and the circumstances of the urine loss. For example, you may have leaked with coughing or sneezing (stress incontinence), when unable to get to the toilet in time (urge incontinence), when laughing or giggling or even when asleep. Do not be too bashful or ashamed to write down what is happening to you. Only by keeping a record of what your bladder is doing will you make progress and be encouraged to go on making progress. Keep your old charts to remind you of how bad you were when you first started.

Do continue to keep your time and volume chart daily to see for yourself what progress you are making throughout the whole of the 3-month programme.

TIME AND VOLUME RECORD

NAME: ....

DATE	TIME	INTERVAL	VOLUME	LEAKAGE
2 JAN	7.0 am		180	WET
	8.0	1 HR	50	
	8.45	3/4 HR	60	
	9.15	1/2 HR	40	URGE
	10.30	1 1/4 HR	90	
	12.0	1 1/2 HR	110	
	1.0 pm	1 HR	20	FLOOD!
	1.45	3/4 HR	40	URGE WASHING UP
	3.0	1 1/4 HR	90	
	4.30	1 1/2 HR	100	
	6.0	1 1/2 HR	80	
	6.45	3/4 HR	50	URGE WATER RUNNING
	8.0	1 1/4 HR	70	
	9.15	1 1/4 HR	90	
	10.30	BED 1 1/4 HR	100	
	2.0 am	3 1/2 HR	120	
	4.30	2 1/2 HR	90	
3 JAN	7.15	2 3/4 HR	170	WET AGAIN
	8.15	1 HR	60	
	9.30	1 1/4 HR	100	

Figure 5: Example of a time and volume chart from a severely affected individual with an unstable bladder. Note frequent voiding and small bladder capacity by day. Incontinence occurs with running water and on getting out of bed in the morning as well as at other times. Even though the bladder will hold 120ml, most of the time only half this capacity is used.

TIME AND VOLUME RECORD

NAME: ....

DATE	TIME	INTERVAL	VOLUME	LEAKAGE
4 APR	7.0am	8 HR	520	
	12.0	5 HR	400	
	4.30pm	4½ HR	380	
	8.30	4 HR	430	
	11.0	2½ HR	210	
5 APR	7.0am	8 HR	580	
	11.30	4½ HR	350	
	4.30pm	5 HR	410	
	9.0	4½ HR	390	
	10.30	2½ HR	190	
6 APR	7.15am	8 ¾ HR	600	DRY!
	11.45	4½ HR	450	
	4.15pm	4½ HR	320	
	7.30	3¼ HR	310	
	11.0	3½ HR	290	
7 APR	7.0am	8 HR	490	
	11.45	4¾ HR	370	
	4.30pm	4¾ HR	430	

Figure 6: Typical time and volume chart of the same woman 3 months later. Note that the bladder capacity has increased markedly and that even with a volume of 600ml the patient is dry. This sort of improvement is common in people who follow the bladder training programme carefully. Both bladder capacity and control will return to normal with persistence.

In filling in the chart be honest, be accurate, be consistent and be intelligent. Try to compare the volume you measure with the volume you thought was in the bladder when it signalled it was full. You will notice that very often it can feel fuller with a small volume than with a large one. Notice that the urine is often more irritant when it is dark in colour than when it is paler. Notice how often your bladder tells lies about how full it is. Try to relate small volume voids to specific incidents or events which provoked them; for example, showering, having bowels open, anxiety or whatever. Find out by trial and error whether coffee, tea or alcohol provoke your bladder to misbehave.

Try to distinguish between different bladder sensations. The unstable bladder, when it contracts gives rise to an urgent, knee-crossing, eye-watering desire to urinate even though the bladder may not be full. Note that this sensation is experienced in the region of the urethra – either in the penis in men or 'down below' in women. This sensation is quite different to the 'full' sensation that you get when the bladder is really full, but is not contracting. The 'full' sensation is generally felt in the lower part of the tummy just above the pubic hair.

Get used to these different sensations and learn to distinguish accurately between when your bladder is full and when it is merely being irritable and overactive and lying to you. The bladder is a dreadful liar, but with practice your brain will learn to keep it under control. Consciously tell your bladder to 'shut up' when it is irritating you at a time when it is not full.

Fluid Intake

Start drinking more every day. You should aim to increase your fluid intake up to 2 litres (3½ pints) every day. This means you will have to drink 10 or 12 full cups or glasses of liquid a day. Don't count soup or the milk that you put on morning cereals. In summertime you may need to drink more than this. Aim to get your urine looking the same colour as gin, or at least pale lemon yellow.

Do most of your drinking in the morning and early afternoon. Do not drink anything within 2 hours of going to bed if you want a quiet night. You may drink any kind of liquid you like as long as it isn't fattening. Water is very good but many people find it rather insipid to drink alone. Try flavouring it with low-calorie cordial. Avoid all alcohol as this has a harmful effect on the bladder.

Some people find that their unstable bladders are much more overactive when they drink tea or coffee. The caffeine in these beverages (and in cola) may affect your bladder. You should find out by trial and error whether you are sensitive to caffeine. If you are, you should try the decaffeinated beverages for a while until you start to make progress.

The important point is that you must drink more each day and keep on drinking more. You may find drinking 2 litres (3½ pints) of fluid difficult at first, but do try. People who say that they cannot do it are just not trying, and have the wrong mental attitude. It can be done. It may be that over the years your stomach has become used to only dealing with small quantities of liquid in just the same way as your bladder has. With effort and determination you can change both. Just give it time and keep trying.

The Training Programmes

Two types of bladder training programmes have been used and are detailed below. Both involve trying to increase the amount of urine the bladder will hold. Read through both programmes and choose the one you think will be best for you. Most people tend to choose the timed deferment programme first and then move on to the other technique as they make progress. Having read through the programme of your choice, you will need to work through the section on 'deferment techniques' (page 70) and start practising them before you actually commence your training schedule.

Timed Deferment Programme

This technique of training involves trying to increase the effective capacity of the bladder by 'stretching' it. Instead of going to the toilet as soon as yet get the 'call of nature', you should wait for 5 minutes before going, **each and every time** you get the desire to void.

You may not at first be able to defer micturition by 5 minutes every time you want to go. Perhaps you can only manage 2 or 3 minutes. That doesn't matter. Each person has to start somewhere. What does matter is that you try to do it **every** time you feel the urge to empty the bladder, and record on the time and volume chart the number of minutes that you managed to 'hold on'.

A word or two of warning is appropriate at this point. Firstly, don't try to hold on for too long at first. It is better to hold on for 4 minutes and to get to the toilet dry than to hold on for 5 minutes and get wet. You must learn to walk before you can run! And talking about running, the watchword is **don't**. Get yourself out of the habit of running to the toilet. Most of the time it doesn't help because you can't concentrate on keeping your bladder under control and you therefore get wet anyway. It is much better to try to get your bladder back under your control, and then glide to the toilet with dignity.

At first, don't worry if the increased fluid that you are drinking causes you to have to empty your bladder just as frequently as before you started. As you continue the volume that your bladder will hold will increase and the frequency will diminish as the bladder becomes less overactive and unstable. Give it time and keep watching the volumes. You are in training and it does involve some effort. **Concentrate on improving your bladder capacity.**

You will need to learn some of the deferment techniques (page 70). As you proceed you should aim to slowly increase the period of deferment from 5 to 10 minutes each time, and then from 10 to 20 or 30 minutes. During the time you are putting off going to the toilet you are learning how to suppress the bladder contractions and by filling the bladder with more urine, stretching the wall so it will hold more.

During this time you **must** stop going to the toilet 'just in case'. This is vital because going 'just in case' encourages your bladder to hold only small quantities. The only time you should empty the bladder is when your bladder is full and after you have done your 'hold on' exercise. The exceptions to this rule are last thing at night before going to bed and when the bladder wakes you during the night.

Get out of the habit of blaming your bladder and of telling yourself that you can't do it. Your bladder is simply a muscular bag designed to hold urine. It does not have a mind of its own, despite what you may think. It does what you let it do or what you tell it to do. The more you give in to it and tell yourself that there is nothing you can do about it, the longer you will have trouble. Never say you can't, say you'll try. You may be surprised by what you will achieve given time and determination.

Let's summarize this programme to make it easier to follow:

1. Keep a time and volume chart of how your bladder works **every day.**
2. Increase your fluid intake to **2 litres (3½ pints)** each day.
3. Stop going to the toilet 'just in case'.
4. Put off emptying the bladder for 5 minutes **every** time you get the desire to void.
5. Aim to slowly increase the amount of urine your bladder will hold without leaking by increasing the interval between visits to the toilet.
6. Set yourself a higher target bladder capacity to aim for each week or so.
7. Do not fight your bladder if it wakes you at night. Get up and

empty it and get back to sleep. The night-time problem will disappear when your bladder capacity by day is regularly over 300ml (14fl oz). Avoid drinking within 2 hours of going to bed.
8. Don't give up!

Minimum Voiding Time Programme

This type of bladder training relies upon stretching the bladder by going to the toilet only at rigidly fixed intervals. After you have filled out a time and volume chart as a baseline, set yourself a time interval to aim at. Most people with an unstable bladder problem start off voiding only 50 to 100ml (3 to 5fl oz) of urine every hour or less. If this is you, aim to start off with a time interval of 1½ hours or 2 hours. As with the previous programme, you should increase your fluid intake to 2 litres (3½ pints) of liquid every day.

You should now aim to empty your bladder at the set time interval, and **never** before that time. If you can't manage to last out the full time interval, do at least try, but don't exceed what you are capable of holding in your bladder. You will need to use the deferment techniques outlined on page 70 when you get the urge to void in order to stay in control. This programme can be more difficult to do than the previous programme and if you have trouble coping with this just return to the timed deferment programme and stick with it.

If you choose this programme in preference to the deferment programme it is important to remember to space your drinks out evenly through the day. The effect of this will be that your kidneys will then produce a more or less even flow of urine into the bladder without wide fluctuations which make this type of programme so difficult to follow. As your bladder expands, the time interval should be increased. Generally you should aim to increase the interval between urination by half an hour each week until you regularly can last between 3 and 4 hours, which is the normal voiding interval. By then your bladder should be capable of holding 300 to 400ml (14 to 18fl oz) or more. Do not try to get your bladder capacity up to this figure too quickly because you will almost certainly have difficulty getting to the toilet in time and will lose your self-confidence. Take it slowly but keep trying to improve.

Obviously it is easy to cheat during this programme by not drinking, thus managing to hold on for 4 hours by only having a small quantity in the bladder. The aim of this programme is exactly the same as that of the timed deferment programme above, namely to stretch the bladder in a progressive fashion. You should read the previous section and remember the advice it contains.

Remember also that this programme depends upon you to keep up the challenge to your bladder. It does not matter how quickly or slowly the bladder capacity increases as long as you continue to make a little progress each week. Consistency is also important, and you should try to achieve a chart which shows little variation from day to day, irrespective of the weather. The important thing to aim for is to see the bladder capacity slowly improving week by week with less and less accidents.

To a certain extent both timed deferment and increased interval programmes are complementary. That is to say that most individuals will find benefit from combining the elements of both programmes and this accelerates their progress. Do concentrate on staying dry. It is no good trying to hold 400ml (18fl oz) for 4 hours if you are wet every time.

As both the time interval and bladder capacity improve you will probably notice that you are getting up less often at night. Continue to keep a record of your performance on your time and volume charts.

If you are caring for an elderly relative with an incontinence problem, this type of timed voiding programme may make your job easier. Regular voiding every 2 hours or so, by the clock, can often avoid the accidents that result from waiting until the bladder gives a signal that it is full – too late to get to the toilet in time. One of the programmable alarm wrist watches that are now available can be very helpful in reminding the forgetful elderly to go to the toilet at the right time. Obviously this type of management of the problem is only appropriate for those who, through senility or lack of motivation, are unable to cooperate with the training programmes above. Even under these circumstances, you should try as far as possible to improve how much the bladder will hold, especially if bedwetting occurs. Your doctor may be able to prescribe various drugs to assist in restoring continence in such cases.

Deferment Techniques

This section deals with some of the techniques that can be used to control the bladder. Not every method will help everybody and only practice with a number of them will teach any particular person what works for them.

1. **Pelvic Floor Contraction**. This is what you almost instinctively do to prevent urinary leakage when you get the urgent desire to void. It has several effects. Firstly, it elevates the base of the bladder and closes the sphincter muscles around the urethra and anus. It is the closure of the muscles around the urethra (the distal urethral sphincter mechanism), that prevents urine flow during unstable contractions (or not as the case may be). Secondly the contraction of the pelvic floor and sphincter muscles suppresses the bladder contraction by a reflex in the spinal cord. It does this more quickly and effectively if the pelvic floor contraction is vigorously applied very early on in the course of an unstable bladder contraction before very high pressures are reached. The reflex inhibition of the bladder contraction is also better if the urine never flows and if the 'brake' can be applied with persistence. Obviously if the pelvic floor and sphincter muscles are relaxed before the bladder contraction has gone away, leakage will occur.

   With practice you will find that the muscles get stronger and you will find that the bladder contractions do go away if they meet sufficiently determined resistance. Once the bladder contraction has been suppressed in this way there is no longer any danger of leakage on the way to the toilet. Indeed, at a later stage, you will find that it may be 20 or 30 minutes before you get another desire to void.

   If your pelvic floor or the sphincter muscles are weak you will need to concentrate on the pelvic floor exercise programme in Section 2 of this book, either before you start bladder training or at the same time. In any event you should work through the preparatory pelvic floor exercises at the start of your bladder training programme to make sure that you know which muscles to use to put on the 'brake'. Throughout the rest of the training period you should regularly perform the basic pelvic floor exercises as specified in Section 2 (pages 25-32). Concentrate particularly on the slow sustained contractions in order to build up strength and stamina in the sphincter and pelvic floor muscles. Until you get your sphincter and pelvic floor muscles strong enough to withstand the force of contraction of the bladder you will go on getting occasional leakage.

All the other deferment techniques involve using pelvic floor and sphincter contraction at the same time to prevent leakage from occurring whilst the bladder is still having an unstable contraction. If therefore you relax these muscles before the unstable contraction (and the urgent desire to void that it gives rise to) has gone away, you will get wet.

2. **Perineal Pressure**. This technique may already be known to you. At least you will be familiar with the fact that the bladder is easier to control when you are sitting rather than standing. Pressure on the perineum, especially the area between the vagina and rectum (or the scrotum and rectum in men), reflexly suppresses unwanted bladder contractions. This is not always easy to achieve in daily life however. In practice try sitting on the arm of a chair when you get the desire to void, getting the pressure right in the mid-line between the buttocks and also between rectum and vagina (or rectum and scrotum in men). Augment this by contracting the pelvic floor muscles and concentrate on suppressing the bladder contraction. Sitting on your heel or on the edge of a firm chair may be equally helpful. Don't give up until you feel the bladder contraction has gone, and even then keep the 'brake' on by contracting the pelvic floor and sphincter muscles while you stand up.

3. **Penile Squeeze**. This technique is an extension of what little boys do the whole world over when they are learning to control their bladders. The penis is squeezed between thumb and forefinger just behind the glans or tip. The grip should be firm and applied front to back and not from side to side. This squeeze technique is used to increase the bladder suppression achieved by central control and pelvic floor countraction. It can be applied via the trouser pocket to prevent embarrassment. Don't let go until it is safe to do so.

4. **Mental Distraction**. This is vital to the success of all the techniques and fundamental to the whole training programme. When the bladder contracts to try and empty under inappropriate circumstances, the urgent desire to void brings the toilet to mind almost inevitably. It is important to try to get the mental image of the toilet out of mind by concentrating on something else. It really doesn't matter what you choose to think about. When the time comes try mental arithmetic. Attempt to take 9s or 7s away from 100 − 93, 86, 79, 72, and so on. Often, by the time you have finished, the bladder contraction has gone away. Alternatively try controlled breathing, word games, reciting poetry or whatever you find easy and helpful. Just keep your mind off that toilet!

   Other people find that crossing the legs, clenching the fists very firmly or curling the toes downwards helps to distract them. Try these for yourself and see which helps you most. You must concentrate on the physical action you are performing in order to block out thoughts of going to the toilet. Don't give up until the feeling of needing to empty the bladder has gone away.

5. **Breathing Exercises**. Controlled respiration is really just another type of mental distraction. There are two techniques, shallow panting or controlled slow inspiration and expiration to maximum lung capacity. Try this technique. When you get the desire to urinate, stand still, contract the pelvic floor muscles and then take a slow, deep breath in, really filling the lungs and feeling your chest expand fully − a bit more, then a bit more again. At the same time flatten the lower part of your tummy and hold it in. Now slowly, very slowly breath out, letting your chest sink down again but keeping the tummy drawn in. Let all the air out. Do the whole sequence once more if the feeling in your bladder has not returned to normal after one breathing cycle. Keep the lower part of your tummy drawn in flat and still until it is safe to move on.

   The important point is to concentrate hard on the breathing instead of the bladder. Of course, you will have to put the 'brake' on by contracting the pelvic floor and sphincter muscles, and keep them pulled tight until the bladder contraction dies away.

Any or all of the techniques can be used. It is really a matter of trying them all to see what suits each individual. Repetition and determination are the keys to success. At first you may find it safer to run to the toilet and then practise the deferment techniques there. This is **not** a good idea and you should try to learn how to control the bladder wherever you are rather than giving way to it. The sooner you start to get back in control the better. Stand or sit still when you get that desire to void and get your bladder under control. If you are in the street stop and look in a shop window or at a garden, do your deferment exercise, then walk on dry and triumphant.

Remember to use one or more of these deferment techniques to suppress the unstable bladder contractions **each and every time** you get the urgent desire to urinate. Only by doing this regularly will you learn to regain control over your bladder. It is going to be a hard struggle but it is very worthwhile. Slowly it will become easier and easier to do and you will find that, as the bladder capacity improves, you will have to fight your bladder less often.

Once the intense desire to void has gone away or diminished your bladder may still feel full. If so, go and empty it. If it is not full try to go on with what you were doing before your bladder interrupted you and wait until the next time that you get the signal that your bladder needs emptying. Don't forget to attempt another 5 minute 'hold on' when this occurs. It is only when you are working hard at suppressing the unstable contractions that you are really learning to control the bladder.

If you do get caught out and have to 'make a dash for it' you should take extreme care not to relax your control muscles until you are already sitting on the toilet, otherwise you may have an 'accident'. Once you are there safely do make sure that you thoroughly relax to enable the bladder to empty completely. Don't push and strain – just relax. Do not get into the habit of stopping and starting the urinary flow during voiding. This is very important.

Helpful Additional Measures

Many people find that they need additional help with their bladder training programme. Sometimes this is because they find it difficult to break the bad habits of a lifetime whilst in their home environment. Under these circumstances much can often be achieved by a short period away from home under the supportive guidance of a specialized bladder training centre. There are, however, very few of these at present in the UK. Often great progress is made within a week, so such a referral is well worth considering. Discuss this with your family doctor. Some of the other options are outlined below.

Drug Therapy

Your doctor or specialist may be able to help you by prescribing a variety of drugs for you which have the effect of calming the bladder down. These tend to be more effective in the elderly and in those people in whom the bladder overactivity results from disease of the nervous system – such as spina bifida, multiple sclerosis, Parkinson's disease, spinal injury or after a stroke.

For those with no such obvious cause for bladder instability, such drug treatment is best regarded as a temporary help whilst bladder training is being tried. As there are a large number of drugs which can be helpful you will have to be guided by your medical adviser. Some people are more sensitive to such agents than others and a trial of different agents either alone or in combinations may be necessary. Remember that at best these agents are only going to help you to control your own bladder – they are not going to do it for you.

Biofeedback

Biofeedback is only available at a few centres worldwide but is a very valuable adjunct to conventional bladder training programmes. Biofeedback is a technique in which you are shown what is happening to your bladder in order to help you to gain control over it. It involves filling your bladder up with fluid whilst measuring the pressure inside it. When the pressure rises above normal due to an unstable contraction of the bladder muscle, you will hear a tone which rises in proportion to the rise in the bladder pressure. You may also be able to see the pressure rise causing a column of lights or column of coloured water to rise and fall.

While this is in progress you will be taught some of the deferment exercises above and will see for yourself how effective each is in bringing the pressure inside the bladder back to normal.

As you get better at controlling the bladder you will be asked to do more and more difficult things. In this way you will learn how to keep control whilst getting out of bed, jumping, coughing or being in the presence of running water. The aim is to constantly increase the challenge to your bladder, and to learn to control it even under the worst circumstances.

Biofeedback sessions are conducted at weekly intervals on an outpatient basis normally but more frequently if you are in hospital. Not everybody needs this type of help, and the number of sessions any one individual needs can vary considerably. It is not uncommon to find that patients having biofeedback can hold much more fluid in the bladder during the session than they can when they get home. This does not matter. With time and patience the volume the bladder will hold during normal activity will slowly come close to what you can achieve under supervision.

It is obviously important to put the lessons that you learn during biofeedback into practice during your everyday life. The machine does not do the hard work for you. It is really still up to you to do the exercises. The more effort you put into them the better the result you will get. Nonetheless you may have to be patient and persistent.

Surgical Intervention

The urge incontinence and frequency which results from bladder instability does not respond to the usual 'repair operations' which are often done for the treatment of simple stress incontinence. Indeed, the unstable bladder is the chief cause of failure of such operations to cure incontinence at all ages. There are, however, a number of minor surgical procedures which can help to quieten the unstable bladder. Amongst these, bladder distension and a variety of nerve blocks are the least upsetting and most widely performed.

If your problem is intractable or unresponsive to training along the lines suggested above, you should seek referral to a urologist with a special interest in these matters. An examination of your bladder with a small telescope passed up the urethra under local or general anaesthetic (a cystoscopy) is often advisable to exclude inflammation, stones or tumours in the bladder or obstruction in the urethra.

You should not consent to any 'repair operation' for this type of problem until you have had a urodynamic study and cystoscopy to elucidate the precise cause of your bladder problems. Do not be talked into believing that a cystocoele or prolapse of the bladder base is the cause of your frequency, urgency and leakage. A degree of cystocoele is exceptionally common in women after the menopause and surgical repair of it seldom if ever alleviates the symptoms of the unstable bladder. Similarly, your bladder problem is almost certainly not due to your needing a hysterectomy. Be warned.

Acupuncture

Some continence clinics have found that acupuncture can help patients who are undergoing bladder training. This is experimental at present and you should avoid rushing off to an acupuncture centre in the hope of an instant cure – you will only be wasting your time and money. At best it is only an additional measure to help you with your bladder training programme. It doesn't do the hard work for you.

Making Progress

As you proceed with your bladder training schedule you may find that there are times when you seem to slip backwards. Don't get discouraged. It is important not to go back to your old habits. Keep up the fluid intake above all. Try not to get discouraged by setbacks. If you do have a bad day, don't give up and make it a bad week. Start each day afresh with a positive attitude. Your bladder will not give up without a fight, after all the chances are that you have had the problem for years. Basically this is a fight which you, rather than your bladder, must win.

Your progress will depend critically upon how much effort you put into carrying out the exercises and techniques described above. This may require some changes in your lifestyle. Stress and anxiety, either at home or at work, can have drastic effects on the function of the bladder and you may need some help to learn how to deal with these situations without loss of control. Continue to keep a time and volume chart of your bladder function for a full 3 months.

Be sure to enlist the support of your spouse or family right from the start. Let them read this manual so that they understand what is going on and can be supportive. The more help you can get the better. Your friends can also be of help if you will let them – many of them will have the same sort of problem! If possible get a friend to do these exercises with you and have a competition to see who can get their bladder to hold 400ml (18fl oz) first. This will ensure that you both work hard and encourage each other.

Get your spouse or friend to look at your charts once every week. If you have made progress, congratulations are in order. If you didn't try or failed to keep your chart up to date you should have to pay a pre-arranged fine (£2.50 or £5). This will at least ensure that you put in your very best efforts. You don't have to believe that this programme can help you – it does work **if you follow the instructions!**

Above all do not try to cut corners in the programme or cheat. There is no easy way to re-educate your bladder and your determination to see the whole programme through to success is absolutely vital. Failure to keep your records up to date, or forgetting to drink, will not help you whatever excuse you make. People from every type of occupation have already managed to complete this programme successfully. The more you try to bend the rules to suit your lifestyle, the longer it will take to achieve a cure. In general you will have to give the requirements of this training programme **top priority** in your life before you will be rewarded by early and sustained improvement.

As time goes by you will find that it gets easier to keep control of your bladder. Daytime frequency will diminish and you will have to get up at night less and less frequently. There is no point at all in trying to fight the bladder in bed at night. You will only lose sleep by doing so. If your bladder wakes you in the night get up and empty it and get back to sleep. The night time problem will disappear by itself once the bladder is under control during the day and can regularly hold 400ml (18fl oz) of urine, which is about the quantity that most people produce during 8 to 9 hours of sleep.

Building up your self-confidence

As you begin to see some progress, try to get out of the habit of using incontinence pads. These pads are merely safety nets and encourage laziness. The sooner you throw them away the sooner you will put in your best efforts. Obviously there will be times when you feel that you need the confidence that wearing a pad can bring. Try to get over this as it really is an admission of defeat on your part, and it saps your self-confidence.

As your bladder improves you will find a great improvement in your general health and in your self-confidence. Once you stop having leakage, go out and buy yourself a new article of clothing to celebrate. You are encouraged to wear make-up, take a pride in your appearance and hair, and to lose excess weight. There really is no reason to stop thinking of yourself as a woman because of your bladder problem. You will feel better about yourself if you take more trouble over yourself and that will help you to get on top of the problem.

Tackling Specific Problems

Some people experience peculiar difficulty in controlling the bladder under specific stressful or provocative circumstances. Perhaps you have trouble doing the washing up, or when you hear running water, or when you get out of a chair. These special situations require tackling in a specific way which will increase your self-confidence and reduce the anxiety that inevitably surrounds them.

For the sake of an example let us assume that your problem is related to running water. Every time you hear running water you get an urgent desire to empty your bladder and sometimes leak on the way to the toilet.

Obviously the bladder does not have ears and so it cannot hear the water running. The running water is a 'trigger' which fires off your bladder from your brain. You can learn to desensitize yourself by a sensible and graduated series of exercises.

Commence by convincing yourself that you can listen to running water without any problem when you have just emptied your bladder. Try it out next time you urinate. The time after that go and stand by a running tap 20 to 30 minutes after emptying your bladder. No problem? Now try doing it again 45 minutes or 1 hour after passing urine. If you can manage to do this successfully, do the same thing again for several days in a row to convince yourself that you really can do it.

Now increase the time interval by 15 minutes every 2 or 3 days. After 3 weeks you should be able to stand by a running tap without any problem even 2 hours after emptying your bladder. If you do have a problem on one day don't give up. Go back to what you were able to do 3 days previously and convince yourself that you can still do it. Do the same thing for several more days in a row to build up your confidence again. Then try the difficult situation once more. Your sense of triumph on succeeding will be worth the effort.

You have not finished yet. You must go on challenging yourself to do better and better. Now try emptying your bladder, waiting 2 hours, having a drink and then turning on the tap. If you can do that, have a drink of cold water whilst listening to the tap running. Now you really have desensitized your bladder. Don't just do this once or twice and then forget about it, keep practising until you no longer think of it as being something special.

By using the same technique you can learn to keep the bladder under control under all sorts of circumstances which may seem impossible before you try it. Try doing the same thing when you are going out of the house shopping. Start off with a short shopping trip (say half an hour) commencing immediately after emptying your bladder. Next day, do exactly the same trip but start out half an hour after you passed urine. Gradually increase the time interval between emptying your bladder and setting off from home. When you can manage to wait 2 hours before leaving home and can still get home without a problem, change your route so that the trip takes one hour instead of just half an hour, but leave home only one hour after emptying your bladder.

Keep on in this way until you can be away from home and remain dry 3 hours after voiding, then start having a drink before you leave home. After a couple of months you should have built up enough courage and confidence to be able to go shopping with a friend without even stopping to think when it was that you last emptied your bladder. Some people have even got to the stage where having a coffee with friends whilst away from home no longer poses a threat to them. Remember to take it gently. If you have an 'accident', go back to what you could do the week before and restore your self-confidence. Stop wearing pads when you are away from home as soon as you can.

As a final example let's suppose that one of your problems is getting to the toilet without leaking when you first get up in the morning. Many people with unstable bladders have this problem because their bladder is fullest at this time of day. You will first of all have to practise the pelvic floor exercises until you can sustain a contraction, without weakening, for 10 to 20 seconds. Then with an empty bladder, practise getting out of bed keeping the pelvic floor fully contracted. Whilst lying in bed, put on the 'brake', slowly sit up and swing your legs onto the floor and stand up carefully. With the 'brake' still on see if you can walk to the toilet and sit down before you relax the pelvic floor muscles. Keep practising this **during the day with an empty bladder** until you can do it easily. Now practise the same thing, again during the day, with more and more urine in the bladder. In the end you will be good enough to do it every morning. It isn't going to be easy, but the problem won't get better until you try to do something about it.

Remember always to 'put on the brake' **before** you start to do something which might be likely to provoke your bladder. In this way you can prevent the bladder from contracting in the first place, instead of having to fight it once it has contracted.

These 3 examples of how to tackle problem areas of bladder control should help you to devise a graduated approach to your own individual difficulties. Your unstable bladder is not going to go away by itself. Once you have started to make progress with the basic training programme you should take courage and map out a plan for coming to grips with the situations in life that currently make you lose control.

Writing down when you leak on a chart is extremely valuable in these sorts of circumstances. By doing so you clearly identify the areas of your life and activities that cause the most problem. Meet these head on. If you don't tackle them now they will plague you for the rest of your life.

Disturbed Nights

Getting up at night to pass urine (called nocturia) can be very persistent. About 33% of the population get up once at night to empty the bladder. This is particularly common in the elderly and those who sleep lightly. Many people find that it is difficult to get back to sleep if they do wake at night without first emptying the bladder, but this is seldom a problem.

When the need to pass urine results in 2, 3 or more visits to the toilet during the night, bladder training can be effective in reducing the problem by increasing the effective bladder capacity. However, nocturia is often the last thing to improve. On our bladder training programme most people find that they cannot sleep through the night until the daytime bladder capacity is between 300 and 400ml (14 to 18fl oz) consistently.

In elderly men, nocturia of recent onset may be caused by enlargement of the prostate gland. If this is the case there will usually be other symptoms of obstruction to the bladder outlet – diminished rate of flow, delay in starting, dribbling or incomplete emptying. A simple test of the rate of urine flow during urination (flow rate) will quickly determine whether obstruction is present or not. Once any obstruction is removed, the bladder will either settle down spontaneously over a period of weeks or months, or will then respond to a training programme.

Unfortunately, some people with the nocturia problem pass considerably more urine than 400ml (18fl oz) during the course of the night and so they still have to get up despite good bladder control by day. Examine your time and volume chart and work out how much urine you pass between going to bed and having breakfast. If it is over 600ml (27fl oz) in total you will probably go on having disturbed nights. There may be a reversible cause for this high volume of urine production.

1. Excessive fluid intake – especially just before retiring to bed. Cut out the 'nightcap' and try to avoid drinking within 2 hours of going to bed. Alcohol and coffee are particularly to be avoided because they are diuretics – they stimulate urine production.

2. Reabsorption of retained fluid. If you suffer from swollen ankles or legs, for whatever reason, the body is retaining fluid. This fluid accumulates in the tissues of the lowest parts – ankles, legs, thighs and fingers – under the influence of gravity. During the night when you are lying down, the fluid is reabsorbed into the blood stream. This dilutes the blood and stimulates the kidneys to produce more urine in order to eliminate the excess fluid.

    There are many causes for this fluid retention. Try cutting down on your intake of salt. Put your feet up in the afternoon or in the evening when you are sewing or watching television. Consult your family doctor and have him check you over to exclude a serious problem. If he suggests a diuretic drug ('water pills') ask him to avoid the fast-acting ones as this may give you a problem during the day! Try to avoid the long-term use of these agents if you can, especially if you only have a minor problem around period time.

3. Failure of normal nocturnal urine concentration. The kidneys normally shut down urine production during the night under the influence of various hormones. During the night the urine that is produced is concentrated and therefore deeply coloured. If the urine you produce at night is not noticeably darker than it is during the daytime, you may have a kidney problem. If drinking less does not result in you producing a darker-coloured urine at night with a lower volume of output, consult your doctor without delay.

    In the elderly the kidney does lose some of its ability to concentrate the urine as part of an overall deterioration in its function. Sometimes nothing much can be done about this and nocturia then just has to be accepted. Nonetheless, improving the bladder capacity by training will still reduce the amount of trouble you have at night and is well worthwhile.

Maintaining Your Progress

Even if your bladder shows improvement after only a few weeks, you must continue with your training programme for a **full 3 months.** This will ensure that you consolidate your bladder control and that the exercises you have been doing become almost automatic. At this time most people will have made considerable progress, or be completely cured. This is the time to get out the first time and volume chart that you filled in and compare it with your most recent chart.

Most people fall into one of 3 categories at this stage:

1. Cured – full control, no frequency, good capacity.
2. Almost perfect – occasional frequency or rare accidents.
3. Little or no progress – still wet with frequency and urgency.

What you do at the end of your 3-month training programme will depend upon which of these categories you fall into.

Category 1 – Cured. If the programme has worked for you, you will probably have worked very hard to achieve this. Congratulations! It is very important not to slip backward during the coming months and years. In order to prevent this you should keep up your fluid intake – forever. Most people with normal bladders drink 1.5 to 2 litres (3 to 4 pints) of fluid each day and you should do so too. You can, however, stop keeping a time and volume chart every day. We recommend that you 'spot check' your bladder capacity once or twice a week for the next 3 months to make sure that your bladder remains stretched. Keep doing the pelvic floor exercises to keep your control muscles in trim. During the next year continue to occasionally check your bladder volume. If the volumes diminish, put yourself back on to regular measurement until your bladder capacity improves once more.

Category 2 – Significant improvement but not perfect. Obviously you have been doing the right things but you may need more time. It doesn't matter how long it takes to achieve full bladder control as long as you are making progress each week. If this is the case with you, just continue with your bladder training for a few months longer. If at the end of this time you are cured or have only very rare problems proceed as outlined under the Category 1 heading.

If, on the other hand, you are still not satisfied with the outcome you have achieved you should seek professional help from your doctor or a specialist. It is highly likely that you need extra help of some kind. It is probable that, with the right kind of help from a specialist or a continence clinic, you will achieve a good result. Don't give up at this stage.

Category 3 – Little or no improvement. The first thing you should ask yourself is whether you really followed the programme instructions. The chief cause of failure to improve is failure to really try. If you didn't keep charts, forgot to drink enough, or just gave up after a couple of weeks you have no-one to blame but yourself. Start again.

If you really did put in your best efforts and still are no better, you will need full investigation of your bladder problem by a specialist with an interest in this problem. Get your urine checked for infection and talk to your family doctor about the best specialist to see in your area. The sooner you do this the better. The problem will not go away by itself and you need the best advice and help that you can get.

Conclusion

This bladder training programme has revolutionized the lives of 75% of the women, and 60% of the men who have **completed** the full 3-month course. There is no reason why it can't also help you with your bladder problem. It does take time, and a great deal of effort and determination, but you must follow the instructions carefully and complete the course. It is well worth that effort as many people will attest.

The techniques that are contained in this manual may be quite new to many family doctors and your own doctor may be amongst these. If you do have cause to consult him whilst you are on one of these programmes it would be wise to take this manual along with you so that he can see it.

The author wishes you every success in your effort to regain control over your bladder. If you come across some special 'trick' that helps you get control of your bladder that is not mentioned in this manual, the author would like to hear about it. None of us is too old to learn new tricks! Again, it is now up to you. Good luck!

Section Four

Other Types of Incontinence

After-dribble

The loss of a few drops of urine on leaving the toilet after urinating is a problem which mainly affects men. It is epitomized by the somewhat impolite but accurate saying 'no matter how many times you shake it, the last drop always goes down the trouser leg'. This type of leakage afflicts men of all ages.

When there are no other urinary problems it is not a sign of serious significance. What is happening is that the urethra is not being emptied completely by the muscles surrounding it. The best way to eliminate this problem is to 'milk' these last drops from the urethra with a finger before giving the final shake.

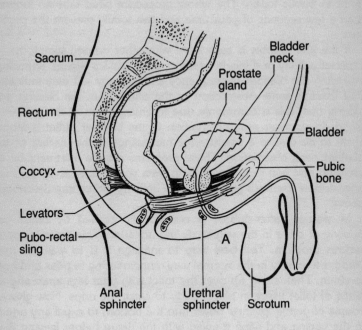

Figure 7: Side view of the male pelvic floor and pelvic organs.

The technique is as follows. After passing urine wait a few seconds for the bladder to empty completely. Place the fingertips of the left hand on the perineum 3 finger-breadths behind the scrotum and apply gentle pressure (see figure 7, point A).

Keeping the pressure in the mid-line gently but positively draw the fingers forward towards the base of the penis, under the scrotum. This milks the urine from the back end of the urethra forward into the anterior or penile urethra from where it can be emptied by shaking or squeezing in the usual way. Repeat the exercise twice to ensure complete emptying of the whole urethra before leaving the toilet.

With practice at home this technique can be performed discretely with a hand in the trouser pocket to prevent embarrassment in public toilets. The whole procedure need take no longer than a few seconds of your time and can totally prevent the problem.

If the after-dribble is associated with other urinary symptoms – especially delay or difficulty starting, poor urinary stream, difficulty emptying the bladder or frequency and urgency – it may indicate that there is some obstruction to the outlet from the bladder. In elderly men this is commonly due to enlargement of the prostate gland. In younger men obstruction to the bladder outlet is more likely to be due to a stricture (or narrowing) of the urethra or to bladder neck obstruction. These problems require treatment by a urologist and you should seek help from your doctor. Even so, the after-dribble itself will respond to the 'milking' procedure described above.

In women, after-dribble is occasionally caused by reflux or pooling of urine in the vagina during urination. This again is not a serious problem. The best way to manage it is to wait for the bladder to empty in the normal way, remembering to relax and not to strain. Then stand up over the toilet with your legs apart and a piece of toilet tissue in place ready to catch the drips. Now give a couple of gentle 'pushes' down into the bottom to expel any urine in the vagina and wipe it away with the tissue before leaving the toilet.

Overflow Incontinence

When the bladder does not empty properly for any of a variety of reasons, the amount of urine left in the bladder is called the **residual urine.** If the condition is progressive and is not treated, larger and larger amounts of residual urine are left in the bladder and result in stretching of the bladder wall. The combination of this retained urine and distension of the bladder wall may cause the neck of the bladder to be pulled open and thus become 'leaky'.

When this occurs all types of incontinence may result – stress incontinence (with coughing, straining or exercise), urge incontinence, and quiet, dribble incontinence without provocation or warning. This whole condition is known as **overflow incontinence** because it is associated with a distended bladder. Up to 15% of elderly women with incontinence have this type of problem. The constant residual urine may result in recurrent infections and the distended bladder may cause lower abdominal swelling.

The effective management of this type of problem depends upon accurate assessment and elimination of the cause of the failure of bladder emptying. In men this may mean an operation to remove obstruction to the bladder outlet. In either sex, subtle or overt damage to the nerve supply to the bladder, diabetes, drugs or nervous tension can result in this type of bladder failure. Clearly this warrants referral to a specialist.

If the bladder cannot be made to empty satisfactorily by itself, your specialist may suggest that you learn how to empty it intermittently by a catheter. A catheter is a small plastic or metal tube which you can insert through the urethra to empty the bladder 3 or 4 times a day. Often this type of management results in complete cessation of the leakage problem as well as eradicating infections.

The technique is very easy to learn and most people pick it up in 2 days or so. All that is required is 2 good hands and proper instruction. Although many people are horrified at first, the technique has revolutionized the lives of thousands of people throughout the world – young and old, male and female. It is certainly better than having a permanent catheter in the bladder which brings its own problems. Sometimes after a few weeks or months the bladder recovers and begins to empty properly again, at which time the intermittent catheter technique can be discontinued.

Continuous Incontinence

A few unfortunate individuals suffer from leakage of urine all the time. In these people a dribble of urine leaks from them day and night with no periods of dryness.

This type of trouble is usually due to an abnormal opening from the bladder or the ureter (the tube from the kidney to the bladder) to the exterior. This abnormal opening is called a fistula. It may be a congenital abnormality, the child being born with a ureter which opens into the vagina instead of the bladder. From birth such children are wet all the time. In older women a fistula between the bladder and vagina may be caused by damage during childbirth, pelvic surgery or radiotherapy for pelvic tumours. Whatever the cause the treatment usually involves surgery.

In the meantime, the intelligent use of incontinence appliances can make all the difference between a totally miserable existence and a reasonably active and tolerable life. The appendix (page 93) contains a guide to the most commonly used appliances for men and women. Some home nursing services have nurse continence advisers who can visit your home to give advice on promotion of continence and show you what is available in the way of appliances. Don't be too shy or embarrassed to ask for help. Your family doctor should be able to put you in touch with suitable advice if you don't know where to start looking for help in your area.

Appendix

Incontinence Appliances

1. For minor degrees of incontinence

Most people with only small volume leakage find that normal feminine hygiene pads or panty liners are sufficient protection. There are a large number on the market from which to choose. Select one to suit your needs.

2. For moderate degrees of incontinence

When leakage is either more frequent in occurrence or of larger volume, or when you know that you are going to be doing something strenuous, a more substantial form of protection may be required. A heavier feminine hygiene product, such as the 'super' pads, is appropriate.

3. For severe incontinence

If leakage is severe and frequent you will need a pad capable of absorbing a large amount of urine, or a specially designed protective undergarment. The range to choose from is limited.

Softeze Dri-Shields Pads. These are bulky pads with a good absorptive capacity. They can be worn inside your own underwear or in specially designed pants such as Dri-shields stretch pants, Softeze brief or the Urocare Incontinence Pants. Obtainable from pharmacies and supermarkets.

Depend Undergarment. This is a new product incorporating a sophisticated absorptive material in a disposable undergarment suitable for most sizes. It is discrete and holds a considerable amount of urine without wetting the skin. Obtainable from most good pharmacies.

Tranquility Pads and Briefs. Stretch briefs in different sizes which secure 'gel-absorbent' disposable pads in place. These are available by mail-order only — ask your doctor.

4.   For Men

For men with incontinence problems of a mild to moderate nature the Conveen range of products is well worth asking your doctor or your local health clinic about.

For more severe or intractable incontinence problems a variety of latex pubic-pressure urinals is available. Male incontinence devices are available on prescription from your G.P.

5.   For bed protection

When wet beds become a problem the use of a rubber or plastic undersheet will protect the mattress. Alternatively consider obtaining Kylie sheets. These quilted, launderable sheets absorb up to 2500ml of urine. Because the urine is absorbed, the skin is kept drier and is less prone to fungal infection and ulceration. Available from Nicholas Labs. Ltd., 225 Bass Road, Slough, Berkshire, 0753 23971. Disposable bed pads are available from the District Nursing Service if the laundry presents a problem.

Glossary

Abdomen The abdomen is the medical term for the belly or tummy and extends from the diaphragm and rib cage at the top, down to the pelvis. Its contents include the gut (stomach, duodenum, small bowel and large bowel), liver, spleen, pancreas and kidneys – collectively known as the abdominal organs – all within one cavity, the abdominal cavity.

Anus The anus is the terminal segment of the bowel. Commonly called the 'back passage', it is surrounded by sphincter muscles allowing control over the passage of wind (flatus) and motions (faeces).

Bladder The bladder is a muscular bag designed to store urine and to expel it under voluntary control. It is situated in the pelvis and lies behind the pubic bone and in front of the vagina and rectum (see figure 1).

Bladder neck The neck of the bladder lies at the base of the bladder itself and at its exit into the urethra. It is normally closed and watertight and opens only when the bladder contracts in order to empty. If it is damaged it may no longer be watertight and stress incontinence may occur with coughing, straining or exercise.

Coccygeus One of the levator group of muscles of the pelvic floor (see figure 2).

Coccyx The coccyx is the 'tail bone' and can be felt just behind the anus. It is the human equivalent of the tail of lower animals (see figures 1 and 3).

Congenital abnormality A defect or abnormality of development existing at or from birth.

Continence adviser A health professional, usually a nurse, who has specialist knowledge of prevention and management of incontinence, and promotion of continence.

Cystocoele A cystocoele is a condition in which the base of the bladder drops downwards towards the vulva. It is caused by weakness of the tissues and muscles which normally support the bladder within the pelvis. Many women who have had 2 or more children develop this condition after the menopause. Although it is common it very rarely causes any bladder symptoms and unless it is gross it seldom warrants surgical treatment.

Cystoscopy A visual examination of the interior of the bladder using a small telescope passed up the urethra under local or general anaesthesia.

Detrusor muscle This is the name given to the muscle in the wall of the bladder.

Fistula An abnormal opening between two or more organs. For example, between bladder or ureter and vagina, rectum or skin.

Genitals Sexual organs which are visible between the legs.

Hysterectomy The surgical removal of the uterus (womb). It may be performed through the abdomen (abdominal hysterectomy) or through the vagina (vaginal hysterectomy).

Ilio-coccygeus One of the levator group of pelvic floor muscles (see figure 2).

Incontinence Incontinence is the involuntary loss or escape of urine from the bladder causing 'wetting' or 'leakage'. When this occurs in response to sudden activity such as coughing, sneezing, straining or exercise it is called stress incontinence. When it occurs in association with a strong desire to void it is called urge incontinence. When it occurs without provocation or warning it is called 'quiet' or dribble incontinence.

Labia The name given to the fleshy folds of skin surrounding the opening to the vagina and forming part of the vulva. Sometimes known as the 'lips' of the vagina.

Levators The collective term for the muscles of the pelvic floor which support the abdominal and pelvic organs.

Menopause The menopause is the medical term for the 'change of life'. It is the time in a woman's life when the periods cease and is associated with various hormonal changes. It usually occurs between 45 and 55 years of age.

Menstruation The medical term for 'periods' in which the lining of the womb is shed together with a variable amount of blood in response to hormonal changes.

Micturition The voluntary act of passing urine to empty the bladder at an appropriate time and place.

Perineum The perineum is the 'saddle area' between the legs (see figure 3). Its midpoint is the perineal body lying between the vagina and anus.

Prolapse A prolapse is a condition in which there is descent of the pelvic organs due to weakening of the supporting ligaments and muscles. Usually it refers to descent (or dropping) of the uterus down into the vagina. This may, or may not, be associated with descent of the bladder (cystocoele) and/or the rectum (rectocoele). It generally gives rise to a 'dragging' sensation within the pelvis and may cause actual pain. When it is gross it can cause bladder symptoms.

Prostate The prostate gland is only present in men. It lies just below the neck of the bladder and surrounds the urethra at this point. The gland produces a fluid which forms a large part of the semen. With advancing years the gland may enlarge and cause obstruction to the flow of urine by compression of the urethra. (See figure 7).

Pubo-coccygeus One of the larger of the levator group of pelvic floor muscles (see figure 2).

Pubo-rectalis Part of the levator group of muscles originating at the pubic bone at the front and sweeping backward around the junction between the rectum and anus. At this point it forms a sling supporting the rectum and takes some part in bowel control. See figure 2.

Rectum The rectum is the lower dilated portion of the large bowel. It lies in the pelvis in front of the sacral bone and behind the bladder and vagina. It empties to the exterior via the anus.

Scrotum The scrotum is the sac which holds a man's testicles.

Sphincter A sphincter muscle is a circular band of muscle surrounding any tube in the body on which it may act as a 'valve' to regulate the passage of fluids or solids through that tube. Sphincters exist around the exit from the stomach, around the anus and around the urethra as well as many other areas.

Stable bladder The stable bladder only contracts when the bladder is emptied under full voluntary control and does not contract at any other time. (Compare with unstable bladder). It is the normal bladder behaviour of adults. It requires that the owner has a normal nervous system, motivation to be continent and proper bladder training in childhood.

Unstable bladder The unstable or overactive bladder is one which contracts to try to empty inappropriately during filling or in response the provocation, giving rise to a strong and very urgent desire to pass urine. People with this type of bladder behaviour have to void frequently and urgently by day and often get up several times at night to empty their bladders. In children it is a common cause of bedwetting and daytime urgency such that the child always seems to 'leave it until the last minute'. In infancy it is normal but disappears as toilet training succeeds in teaching the toddler bladder control, the bladder then becoming 'stable'. In adults, instability may be caused by disease of the nervous system, obstruction to the urethra (as occurs with enlargement of the prostate gland), or secondary to severe inflammation of the bladder. Most commonly in women no particular cause is found.

Uterus The uterus is the medical term for the womb.

Ureter The ureters are thin muscular tubes which run from the kidneys on each side down to the bladder. Muscular action in the ureters actively propels urine from kidney to bladder and is independent of gravity — allowing the bladder to fill when we are lying flat or even upside down!

Urethra The urethra is the tube leading from the bladder to the exterior. In the female it is about 4 to 5 centimetres (1½ to 2 inches) long and surrounded by the urethral sphincter mechanism. In the male it is longer and extends through the whole length of the penis. Just below the bladder neck of the male it passes through the prostate gland (enlargement of which may cause obstruction to the flow of urine) and then through the sphincter mechanism before entering the base of the penis.

Urethral sphincter The urethra is surrounded by a sphincter mechanism which acts as a control 'valve'. It is made up of several different types of muscle arranged broadly in a circular fashion around the urethra in such a way as to constrict the urethra to slow down or stop the flow of urine down the urethra from the bladder. The pressure that these muscles exert on the urethra is called the urethral closure pressure and as long as this pressure remains above the pressure inside the bladder no urine will escape.

Urodynamic study Urodynamic testing is a way of studying the behaviour of the bladder and urethra by measuring the pressures within the bladder and/or the urethra during filling and emptying of the bladder and under mechanical stress. When these pressure tests are combined with x-ray examination at the same time the precise cause of incontinence or voiding difficulties can be diagnosed with certainty.

Urologist A specialist dealing specifically with disorders of the urinary tract.

Voiding The act of emptying the bladder to completion – see also micturition.

Vulva The external genital region of the female.

Index

TIME AND VOLUME RECORD

NAME: ....

DATE	TIME	INTERVAL	VOLUME	LEAKAGE

TIME AND VOLUME RECORD
NAME

TIME AND VOLUME RECORD

NAME: ....

DATE	TIME	INTERVAL	VOLUME	LEAKAGE

TIME AND VOLUME RECORD

NAME: ....

DATE	TIME	INTERVAL	VOLUME	LEAKAGE

TIME AND VOLUME RECORD

NAME: ....

DATE	TIME	INTERVAL	VOLUME	LEAKAGE

TIME AND VOLUME RECORD

NAME: ....

DATE	TIME	INTERVAL	VOLUME	LEAKAGE

TIME AND VOLUME RECORD

NAME: ....

DATE	TIME	INTERVAL	VOLUME	LEAKAGE

TIME AND VOLUME RECORD

NAME: ....

DATE	TIME	INTERVAL	VOLUME	LEAKAGE

TIME AND VOLUME RECORD

NAME: BDS

DATE	TIME	INTERVAL	VOLUME	LEAKAGE
12/5	0730	8½ hrs	400	—
	10 30	3 hr.	250++	—
	1230	2 hr	50 +	
	1630	4 h	80 c	urge/pain
	200	2 hr	25 c	+ urgt
	1 30	250		
	8 30	600		
	1 30	50	250	
	8 00	6½	150	